T0259935

SpringerBriefs in Public Health

Child Health

Series Editor
Angelo P. Giardino, Salt Lake City, UT, USA

SpringerBriefs in Public Health present concise summaries of cutting-edge research and practical applications from across the entire field of public health, with contributions from medicine, bioethics, health economics, public policy, biostatistics, and sociology.

The focus of the series is to highlight current topics in public health of interest to a global audience, including health care policy; social determinants of health; health issues in developing countries; new research methods; chronic and infectious disease epidemics; and innovative health interventions.

Featuring compact volumes of 50 to 125 pages, the series covers a range of content from professional to academic. Possible volumes in the series may consist of timely reports of state-of-the art analytical techniques, reports from the field, snapshots of hot and/or emerging topics, elaborated theses, literature reviews, and in-depth case studies. Both solicited and unsolicited manuscripts are considered for publication in this series.

Briefs are published as part of Springer's eBook collection, with millions of users worldwide. In addition, Briefs are available for individual print and electronic purchase.

Briefs are characterized by fast, global electronic dissemination, standard publishing contracts, easy-to-use manuscript preparation and formatting guidelines, and expedited production schedules. We aim for publication 8-12 weeks after acceptance.

More information about this series at http://www.springer.com/series/10138

Michelle A. Lopez • Elissa Z. Faro
Suzette O. Oyeku • Jean L. Raphael

Disparities in Child Health

A Solutions-Based Approach

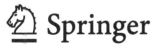 Springer

Michelle A. Lopez
Pediatrics-Hospital Medicine
Baylor College of Medicine
Houston, TX, USA

Suzette O. Oyeku
Division of Academic General Pediatrics
Albert Einstein College of Medicine
Bronx, NY, USA

Elissa Z. Faro
Division of Academic General Pediatrics
Albert Einstein College of Medicine
Bronx, NY, USA

Jean L. Raphael
Pediatrics-Academic General
Baylor College of Medicine
Houston, TX, USA

ISSN 2192-3698   ISSN 2192-3701   (electronic)
SpringerBriefs in Public Health
ISSN 2625-2872   ISSN 2625-2880   (electronic)
SpringerBriefs in Child Health
ISBN 978-3-030-03209-8   ISBN 978-3-030-03210-4   (eBook)
https://doi.org/10.1007/978-3-030-03210-4

Library of Congress Control Number: 2018962001

This Springer imprint is published by the registered company Springer Nature Switzerland AG
The registered company address is: Gewerbestrasse 11, 6330 Cham, Switzerland

Preface

This book was written and co-edited by a group of academic pediatricians who share a common and passionate commitment to addressing the needs of vulnerable populations and ultimately eliminating health disparities among children. Our group strives to untangle the complex and multilayered factors influencing pediatric health disparities. We want others to understand the root causes of inequities in child health and strategies to ameliorate health disparities through clinical care, research, policy, and legislation. The intention of this first edition is to create a state-of-the-art resource for medical students, researchers, clinicians, health policymakers, administrators, and other groups invested in taking a solutions approach to addressing disparities.

Disparities in health and health care have received considerable attention over the past two decades. In 2002, the Institute of Medicine released the landmark report "Unequal Treatment: Confronting Racial and Ethnic Disparities in Health Care." While health disparities as a field has made unprecedented progress, it has largely focused on adults. Less attention has been concentrated toward children.

In this book, readers will find relevant and practical information on the subject of health disparities among children. The objectives of this monograph are to (1) describe how children differ from adults and the relevance to disparities, (2) review current data on pediatric health disparities, (3) provide a framework for addressing disparities among children, (4) describe interventions with the potential to reduce or eliminate health disparities, and (5) outline future avenues for an agenda to address pediatric disparities. Our overarching goal is to provide readers with the tools to successfully engage in addressing pediatric disparities. We truly hope to advance the readers' knowledge and interest in health disparities and child health outcomes. Thank you for your interest in reading our work.

Houston, TX, USA   Michelle A. Lopez
Bronx, NY, USA   Elissa Z. Faro
Bronx, NY, USA   Suzette O. Oyeku
Houston, TX, USA   Jean L. Raphael

Acknowledgments

The authors wish to express their appreciation to:

- Janie Garcia, from the Section of Academic General Pediatrics at Baylor College of Medicine, for her editorial assistance
- Angelo P. Giardino, MD, PhD, MPH, Series Editor, for having the vision to promote critical topics in child health as part of the SpringerBriefs in Child Health Series
- Janet Kim, MPH, Editor, Public Health at Springer, for her consistent encouragement to produce this monograph on Pediatric Health Disparities and offering it as part of the SpringerBriefs in Child Health Series

Contents

1   **Disparities in Child Health: A Review** 1
    Jean L. Raphael and Michelle A. Lopez

2   **Quality of Care in Pediatrics and Health Disparities:**
    The Increasing Role of Quality Improvement Science 11
    Jean L. Raphael, Elissa Z. Faro, and Suzette O. Oyeku

3   **Community Health Worker Interventions** 25
    Michelle A. Lopez

4   **Technology-Based Interventions to Address Pediatric**
    Health Disparities 31
    Michelle A. Lopez

5   **Pediatric Health Disparities and Place-Based Strategies** 39
    Jean L. Raphael

6   **Healthcare Financing and Social Determinants**.................... 47
    Jean L. Raphael

7   **Future Directions for a Solutions-Based Approach** 53
    Jean L. Raphael

Index... 57

Chapter 1
Disparities in Child Health: A Review

Jean L. Raphael and Michelle A. Lopez

Introduction

Since the 2002 publication of the Institute of Medicine's landmark document on health disparities *Unequal Treatment: Confronting Racial and Ethnic Disparities in Health Care*, inequities in the US healthcare system have received unprecedented attention from clinicians, advocacy groups, and policy makers [1]. In Healthy People, a national health promotion and disease prevention initiative, the elimination of health disparities has consistently been listed as an overarching goal [2]. The Agency for Healthcare Research and Quality has issued an annual national health care disparities report since 2003 [3]. In 2010, the National Center on Minority Health and Health Disparities was redesigned as an Institute, elevating the research agenda focused on eliminating health disparities. Researchers, professional organizations, and advocacy groups have made considerable efforts to incorporate addressing health disparities into their strategic goals [4–6].

While health disparities increasingly comprise a focus for health care research, policy, and advocacy regarding adults, little attention is directed towards inequities in children although it is estimated that by 2025, half of all US children with be nonwhite [7]. Comprehensive health reports predominantly focus on adults, with assumptions that the factors contributing to disparities in pediatrics will mirror those of the adult population. In *Unequal Treatment*, only 5 of 103 studies cited specifically addressed disparities in pediatric health care [1]. Over the past decade,

J. L. Raphael (✉)
Pediatrics-Academic General, Baylor College of Medicine, Houston, TX, USA

M. A. Lopez
Pediatrics-Hospital Medicine, Baylor College of Medicine, Houston, TX, USA

the number of research studies addressing pediatric disparities has dramatically increased and covers a wide range of topics, including primary care, inpatient care, and chronic disease management [8–22]. While this outgrowth of research has vastly improved the knowledge around pediatric health disparities, there remains some debate about how to best move forward the discourse on addressing inequities in child health with the goal of innovative solutions-based strategies [23–25]. The goals of this monograph are to (1) describe how children differ from adults and the relevance to disparities; (2) review current data on pediatric health disparities; (3) provide a framework for addressing disparities among children; (4) describe interventions with the potential to reduce or eliminate health disparities; and (5) outline future avenues for an agenda to address disparities in child health.

Definitions

Historically, *disparities* have been defined in the context of differences between racial or ethnic groups (Table 1.1). *Unequal Treatment* defines disparities in health care as "racial or ethnic differences in the quality of health care that are not due to access-related factors or clinical needs, preferences, and appropriateness of intervention." [1] Categories of racial groups include American Indian or Alaska Native, Asian, Black or African-American, Native Hawaiian or other Pacific Islander, and White. Categories for ethnic groups consist of Hispanic or Latino and Not Hispanic or Latino. These definitions have received considerable criticism for several reasons

Table 1.1 Definitions related to health disparities

Term	Source of definition	Definition
Health disparity	Healthy People 2020	Health difference affecting groups of people who have systematically experienced greater obstacles to health based on their racial or ethnic group; religion; socioeconomic status; gender; age; mental health; cognitive, sensory, or physical disability; sexual orientation or gender identity; geographic location; or other characteristics historically linked to discrimination or exclusion
Health equity	Healthy People 2020	Attainment of the highest level of health for all people. Achieving health equity requires valuing everyone equally with focused and ongoing societal efforts to address avoidable inequalities, historical and contemporary injustices, and the elimination of health and health care disparities
Health inequity	World Health Organization	Avoidable inequalities in health between groups of people within countries and between countries. Inequities arise from inequalities within and between societies
Social determinants of health	World Health Organization	The circumstances in which people are born, grow up, live, work and age, and the systems put in place to deal with illness. These circumstances are in turn shaped by a wider set of forces: economics, social policies, and politics

[26–28]. First, the study of racial variation in health care may assume that race is a valid biological category. However, studies have demonstrated that more genetic variation exists within races than between races. Therefore, race has limited biological significance. Second, categorization of racial/ethnic minority groups may fail to reflect how individuals wish to be identified. Third, there are often limitations to how race is measured in most research studies. Methods for collecting race data may vary (e.g., self-report, direct observation, proxy report, and extraction from medical records). Additionally, increasing numbers of individuals belong to multiple racial categories and cannot be classified with a single race category. This increases the challenges in interpreting the influences of race in disparities research.

In addition to race, ethnicity is another variable standardly included in studies on health disparities. The Office of Management and Budget (OMB) includes two ethnic categories in its standards—"Hispanic or Latino" and "Not Hispanic or Latino" and five racial categories: American Indian or Alaska native; Asian; black, or African–American; native Hawaiian or other Pacific Islander; and white [28]. However, like race, defining ethnicity also raises several challenges. The term "Hispanic" includes individuals from over twenty countries who may be diverse in genetics, language, and culture. Children in immigrant families (CIF) are defined as children residing in households with at least one foreign-born parent [29]. Almost ninety percent of them are US citizens. CIF are the fastest growing subset of the US population. The growth of this group is largely driven by births in the Hispanic population. This group experiences unique barriers. CIF are more likely to experience poverty. CIF are more likely to belong to households that are poorly educated. Over 60% of CIF have at least one parent who meets definition for having limited English proficiency.

More recently, researchers and policy makers have expanded the discourse on disparities beyond race and ethnicity in order to acknowledge the diverse set of factors that influence health and health outcomes. Healthy People 2020 defines a *health disparity* as "a particular type of health difference that is closely linked with social, economic, and/or environmental disadvantage [2]. Health disparities adversely affect groups of people who have systematically experienced greater obstacles to health based on their racial or ethnic group; religion; socioeconomic status; gender; age; mental health; cognitive, sensory, or physical disability; sexual orientation or gender identity; geographic location; or other characteristics historically linked to discrimination or exclusion." Increasingly, disparities are framed within the social determinants of health, which are the conditions in the environment in which people are born, live, learn, work, play, worship, and age that impact a wide range of health, functioning, and quality-of-life outcomes [30]. Conditions may be social, economic, or physical. Examples of social determinants include access to health care services, safe housing, schools, neighborhood conditions, built environment, socioeconomic conditions, literacy, and exposure to toxic substances [31].

According to the US Department of Health and Human Services, a *health disparity* is defined by the Health People 2020 description as "a particular type of health difference that is closely linked with social, economic, and/or environmental disadvantage. Health disparities adversely affect groups of people who have systematically experienced greater obstacles to health based on their racial or ethnic group; religion; socioeconomic status; gender; age; mental health; cognitive, sensory, or physical disability; sexual orientation or gender identity; geographic location; or other characteristics historically linked to discrimination or exclusion." As the definition of health disparities has evolved, the concept of health equity has also emerged. According to the World Health Organization, health equity is defined as "the absence of avoidable or remediable differences among groups of people, whether those groups are defined socially, economically, demographically, or geographically. *Health inequities* therefore involve more than inequality with respect to health determinants, access to the resources needed to improve and maintain health or health outcomes. They also entail a failure to avoid or overcome inequalities that infringe on fairness and human rights norms." [30] Implicit in this definition of health equity is that every individual deserves a fair opportunity to lead a healthy life. The concepts of health equity and health disparities are tightly linked in their practical application. Policies and interventions aimed at achieving the goal of health equity will provide a foundation for reducing or eliminating health disparities.

Extrapolating Disparities from Adults to Children

With a large body of research among adult populations documenting disparities across a wide range of conditions and health care services, there is often temptation to assume that children experience disparities as adults do with similar prevalence, conditions, and root causes. However, there is need to consider disparities in pediatrics a distinct field. Pediatric researchers have conceptualized and articulated unique aspects of childhood relative to adults in health services research and policy [32, 33]. These factors consist of development, dependency, differential epidemiology, demographic patterns, and health care financing (Table 1.2). They are commonly referred to as the 5 Ds.

Development

While adult health care primarily focuses on health maintenance and prevention of sequelae associated with disease progression, child health care is predominantly centered on development and well child care. The presentation, clinical course, management, and impact of diseases in childhood are all impacted by development as a child will transitions through multiple developmental stages (infancy, toddler stage, school age, adolescence) towards young adulthood. Small interventions at early stages can dramatically affect long-term outcomes. For example, timely recognition of developmental delay and referral to early intervention services can lead to improved academic success. As children develop cognitive skills over time, their

Table 1.2 5 D's and relevance to disparities

The 5 D's	Child health	Priorities in disparities
Development	• Developmental progress important • Prevention	• Improving access to care • Ensuring equity in content of well child care
Dependency	• Dependent on adults • Parents important • Family health • Critical influences of home environment • Team includes family, school, child care providers	• Addressing social determinants of family • Developing family-focused interventions
Differential epidemiology	• Children mostly healthy • Relatively rare diseases • Specialists in academic institutions	• Improving primary care • Increasing access to care for chronic conditions
Demographics	• High rate of poverty • Increasing numbers of children in immigrant families • Large proportion of racial/ethnic minorities	• Addressing social determinants of health • Incorporating cultural competency into interventions
Dollars	• Diverse set of payers • Health care takes place in numerous settings • Difficult to determine return on investment over the life course	• Tailoring interventions to the different environments in which children receive care • Partnering with Medicaid and CHIP to improve care

potential for self-management vastly increases. They are gradually able to engage more effectively in their own health and health care. In younger stages, they may be completely reliant on adults for managing their health care. During adolescence, children may work collaboratively with their parents. As adolescents become adults, their parents, health care providers, and community must support them as they transition from the child to adult sector. These characteristics have significant implications for health disparities. Careful attention must be paid to the provision of well child care and developmental screening such that there is equity across populations.

Dependency

Children exist within the context of their families and are dependent on parents and other adults for health care. They are also dependent on adults from educational and legal standpoints. Consequently, the health and functioning of the family unit significantly impacts the health and health care of the child. This dependency only has limited parallels in adult health care. For children, parents and the family unit are critical partners in care. As an example, poor physical and mental health of parents adversely impact the health of the child and are associated with increased health care seeking for the child. Therefore, children's dependency requires a broader focus on the entire family. In addition to the family, schools play a key role in the management of health conditions. Consequently, partnerships with the educational sector are critical to promoting child health. Furthermore, as adolescents mature, their role changes and their emerging autonomy must be nurtured. These characteristics generate specific needs as related to health disparities. The social determinants around the family must be adequately addressed in order to maximize health outcomes for all children. Therefore, support services available to families must be robust and comprehensive.

Differential Epidemiology

Relative to adults, children are primarily healthy with the epidemiology of chronic conditions in children somewhat different from what is observed in adults. Aside from a few conditions (e.g., obesity, asthma, mental health disorders), there are fewer concentrations of specific conditions among children. Instead, children may have relatively rare conditions. Given these epidemiologic factors, prevention and routine care may serve as critical targets for intervention. Because of the rarity of chronic conditions in children, most pediatric specialists are based in academic institutions, resulting in limited access to care. These characteristics influence disparities in several ways. First, prevention is critical to address the health needs of all populations. Prevention is especially important for common conditions such as obesity, asthma, and mental health conditions. Second, efforts must be made to increase and ensure access to care such that children with rare conditions from underserved populations have the opportunity to receive comprehensive care.

Demographics

In contrast to adults, children and adolescents have disproportionately high rates of poverty. The pediatric population is also more racially and ethnically diverse. According to the 2010 US Census, racial and ethnic minorities comprise 46% of US children [33]. The combination of poverty and diversity make children particularly vulnerable to poor health and inadequate quality of care. These factors highlight several important priorities with respect to health disparities. First, substantial investment is required to understand and address social determinants of health for children and their families. Second, given the demographics of US children, more efforts must be made to address racial/ethnic and socioeconomic disparities.

Health Care Financing (Dollars)

The financing of child health care differ substantially from that for adults, particularly with respect to individuals with low socioeconomic status. Services for children are provided by a diverse mix of payers, including private insurers, state Medicaid, and Children's Health Insurance Program (CHIP) funds. Adults primarily rely on private insurance and Medicare. In contrast to Medicare, Medicaid and CHIP vary from state to state. They also reimburse providers at 60% of Medicare rates for similar services [33]. While the costs of health care for children are small relative to those for adults, they represent an important investment that may result in savings over the life span. However, policy makers have difficulty in determining the return on investment of spending on children. First, financial benefits may accrue over a much longer period of time relative to adults. Second, savings may occur more in long-term quality of life and less in the medical care system. Financing differences indicate specific needs with respect to health disparities. Since significant numbers of children, specifically those from racial/ethnic minority backgrounds, are insured through Medicaid and CHIP, addressing health disparities requires investment in the quality of care provided through these insurers.

Documented Disparities in Child Health

An extensive body of work has documented that minority children experience lower quality care across the Institute of Medicine's (IOM) dimensions of quality consisting of effectiveness, patient-centeredness, timeliness of care, and patient safety [11, 19]. The evidence for quality gaps according to race/ethnicity has been largely facilitated by periodic population surveys and annually published reports including the National Healthcare Quality Report and National Healthcare Disparities Report funded by the Agency for Healthcare Quality and Research (AHRQ) [34]. Among effectiveness measures, minority children have lower rates of well child visits, family-centered care, weight and height checks during well child visits, counseling, and time alone with providers for teenagers [35, 36]. Among chronic condition management, non-Hispanic black and Hispanic children with asthma are less likely to have daily inhaled anti-inflammatory therapy [12, 37]. For patient-centeredness, minority parents report lower rates of clinical providers listening, explaining things, and spending enough time with regards to their child's care [16]. Among timeliness measures, minority parents are more likely to report difficulty getting appointments for their child when desired. Hispanic children have longer wait times in the emergency care setting relative to other groups [38]. Among patient safety measures, minority children have higher rates of decubitus ulcers and preventable infections during hospitalization [11, 19].

Medical Status

In addition to IOM quality domains, racial/ethnic minority children experience inequities according to other measures. Black and Hispanic children are significantly more likely to be in poor health (not excellent/very good) compared to whites. They are more likely to be overweight/obese. They are also more likely to have conditions such as asthma, attention deficit hyperactivity disorder, depression/anxiety, and behavioral problems [18].

Access to Care and Health Service Use

Relative to white children, black and Hispanic children are significantly more likely to be uninsured and sporadically insured [18]. Compared to whites, black, Hispanic, and American Indian/Alaska Native (AIAN) have greater odds of having no doctor or nurse. In reporting a usual source of care, lower percentages of black (87%) and Hispanic (87%) children have a usual source of care compared to white children (93%). A lower percentage of black (47%) and Hispanic (47%) are reported to have a well-child visit in the last year relative to white children (56%). Parents in all minority groups are more likely to report that that their primary care doctor never/ sometimes spends enough time with the child. Blacks and Hispanic children are more likely to have received no specialty care in the past year. Cumulatively, these studies provide a foundation of work highlighting variability in the care for children.

Disparities According English Proficiency

In addition to race/ethnicity, Limited English Proficiency (LEP) can also act as a source of disparities [18]. Approximately sixteen percent of US Hispanic children live in households led by parents who speak English less than very well. Children in LEP families encounter challenges along the entire continuum of navigating the health care system—accessing care, explaining illness, understanding recommendations and plans of care, and participating in shared decision making. Previous research has demonstrated language barriers to be associated with poor patient safety and quality outcomes, including inadequate management of pain, fewer prescribed medications, medical errors, and overdoses [19].

References

1. Institute of Medicine. Unequal treatment: confronting racial and ethnic disparities in health-care. Washington, D.C.: National Academies Press; 2003.
2. Healthy People. At healthypeople.gov. Accessed 18 Sept 2017.
3. Centers for Medicare and Medicaid Services: State innovation models initiative: general information. At https://innovation.cms.gov/initiatives/state-innovations/. Accessed 10 Aug 2016.
4. Cheng TL, Emmanuel MA, Levy DJ, Jenkins RR. Child health disparities: what can a clinician do? Pediatrics. 2015;136:961–8.
5. Cheng TL, Moon R, Horn I, Jenkins R, Disparities DC-BRCoCH. Introduction: state-of-the-art on child health disparities. Pediatrics. 2015;136:730–1.
6. Braveman P, Barclay C. Health disparities beginning in childhood: a life-course perspective. Pediatrics. 2009;124(Suppl 3):S163–75.
7. Wise PH. Child poverty and the promise of human capacity: childhood as a foundation for healthy aging. Acad Pediatr. 2016;16:S37–45.
8. Beck AF, Huang B, Ryan PH, Sandel MT, Chen C, Kahn RS. Areas with high rates of police-reported violent crime have higher rates of childhood asthma morbidity. J Pediatr. 2016;173:175–82.e1.
9. Beck AF, Klein MD, Schaffzin JK, Tallent V, Gillam M, Kahn RS. Identifying and treating a substandard housing cluster using a medical-legal partnership. Pediatrics. 2012;130:831–8.
10. Beck AF, Simmons JM, Huang B, Kahn RS. Geomedicine: area-based socioeconomic measures for assessing risk of hospital reutilization among children admitted for asthma. Am J Public Health. 2012;102:2308–14.
11. Berdahl T, Owens PL, Dougherty D, McCormick MC, Pylypchuk Y, Simpson LA. Annual report on health care for children and youth in the United States: racial/ethnic and socioeconomic disparities in children's health care quality. Acad Pediatr. 2010;10:95–118.
12. Cabana MD, Lara M, Shannon J. Racial and ethnic disparities in the quality of asthma care. Chest. 2007;132:810S–7S.
13. Chan T, Lion KC, Mangione-Smith R. Racial disparities in failure-to-rescue among children undergoing congenital heart surgery. J Pediatr. 2015;166:812–8.e1–4.
14. Colvin JD, Zaniletti I, Fieldston ES, et al. Socioeconomic status and in-hospital pediatric mortality. Pediatrics. 2013;131:e182–90.
15. Lu MC, Halfon N. Racial and ethnic disparities in birth outcomes: a life-course perspective. Matern Child Health J. 2003;7:13–30.
16. Raphael JL, Guadagnolo BA, Beal AC, Giardino AP. Racial and ethnic disparities in indicators of a primary care medical home for children. Acad Pediatr. 2009;9:221–7.
17. Raphael JL, Zhang Y, Liu H, Tapia CD, Giardino AP. Association of medical home care and disparities in emergency care utilization among children with special health care needs. Acad Pediatr. 2009;9:242–8.
18. Flores G, Committee On Pediatric R. Technical report – racial and ethnic disparities in the health and health care of children. Pediatrics. 2010;125:e979–e1020.
19. Flores G, Ngui E. Racial/ethnic disparities and patient safety. Pediatr Clin North Am. 2006;53:1197–215.
20. Lion KC, Thompson DA, Cowden JD, et al. Impact of language proficiency testing on provider use of Spanish for clinical care. Pediatrics. 2012;130:e80–7.
21. Lion KC, Thompson DA, Cowden JD, et al. Clinical Spanish use and language proficiency testing among pediatric residents. Acad Med. 2013;88:1478–84.
22. Liu SY, Pearlman DN. Hospital readmissions for childhood asthma: the role of individual and neighborhood factors. Public Health Rep. 2009;124:65–78.
23. Raphael JL. Observations from the balcony: directions for pediatric health disparities research and policy. J Appl Res Child. 2013;4.
24. Beal AC, Hasnain-Wynia R. Disparities and quality: the next phase for high-performing pediatric care. Acad Pediatr. 2013;13:S21–2.

25. Homer C. A tall order: improve child health. Acad Pediatr. 2013;13:S5–6.
26. Cook BL, McGuire TG, Zaslavsky AM. Measuring racial/ethnic disparities in health care: methods and practical issues. Health Serv Res. 2012;47:1232–54.
27. Crews DE, Bindon JR. Ethnicity as a taxonomic tool in biomedical and biosocial research. Ethn Dis. 1991;1:42–9.
28. Dehlendorf C, Bryant AS, Huddleston HG, Jacoby VL, Fujimoto VY. Health disparities: definitions and measurements. Am J Obstet Gynecol. 2010;202:212–3.
29. Mendoza FS, Festa NK. New American children: supporting the health and well-being of immigrant populations. JAMA Pediatr. 2013;167:12–3.
30. World Health Organization: Social determinants of health.
31. Neighborhood poverty: context and consequences for children. New York: Russell Sage Foundation.
32. Forrest CB, Simpson L, Clancy C. Child health services research. Challenges and opportunities. JAMA. 1997;277:1787–93.
33. Stille C, Turchi RM, Antonelli R, et al. The family-centered medical home: specific considerations for child health research and policy. Acad Pediatr. 2010;10:211–7.
34. National Healthcare quality and disparities reports.
35. Hambidge SJ, Emsermann CB, Federico S, Steiner JF. Disparities in pediatric preventive care in the United States, 1993–2002. Arch Pediatr Adolesc Med. 2007;161:30–6.
36. Coker TR, Rodriguez MA, Flores G. Family-centered care for US children with special health care needs: who gets it and why? Pediatrics. 2010;125:1159–67.
37. Lieu TA, Lozano P, Finkelstein JA, et al. Racial/ethnic variation in asthma status and management practices among children in managed medicaid. Pediatrics. 2002;109:857–65.
38. James CA, Bourgeois FT, Shannon MW. Association of race/ethnicity with emergency department wait times. Pediatrics. 2005;115:e310–5.

Chapter 2
Quality of Care in Pediatrics and Health Disparities: The Increasing Role of Quality Improvement Science

Jean L. Raphael, Elissa Z. Faro, and Suzette O. Oyeku

Introduction

Despite well documented disparities in health and health care, little is known about what types of interventions have the potential to ameliorate disparities [1]. Many clinical providers, organizations, and policy makers do not know where and how to target efforts towards addressing disparities. Innovate approaches are needed to address health disparities and ensure that every child has access to high quality care. Quality improvement (QI) provides one such approach given its demonstrated effectiveness in improving general outcomes in the health care setting. QI can be defined as "a multidisciplinary, systems-focused, data driven method of understanding and improving the efficiency, effectiveness, and reliability of health processes and outcomes of care" [2]. It consists of continuous actions that aim to measurably improve health care services and the health status of targeted patient groups by improving uptake of evidence-based, best practices into clinical care [3]. Multiple QI frameworks exist [2]. Example approaches include Plan, Do, Study, Act (PDSA), Total Quality Management (TQM), Continuous Quality Improvement (CQI), Business Process Reengineering (BPR), rapid cycle change, lean thinking, Six Sigma, and Focus, Analyze, Develop, Execute/Evaluate (FADE). Although the

J. L. Raphael (✉)
Pediatrics-Academic General, Baylor College of Medicine, Houston, TX, USA

E. Z. Faro · S. O. Oyeku
Division of Academic General Pediatrics, Albert Einstein College of Medicine, Bronx, NY, USA

evidence isn't clear on which specific approach works best, all of these models are effective in elucidating a health care organization's current state, determining areas for improvement, designing and implementing a sequential and iterative strategy to achieve improvement, and subsequently collecting data to monitor progress and adjust the strategy as indicated over time [4, 5]. The ongoing process of QI requires four elements: performance goals, performance measures, QI practices, and feedback and reporting.

Rationale for Using QI to Address Disparities in Child Health

QI has the potential to meaningfully address health disparities through a comprehensive set of empirically tested tools with wide use across health systems. A QI intervention can be defined as a change process in health care delivery systems, services, or suppliers for the intended purpose of increasing the likelihood of clinical quality of care, measured by positive health outcomes for individuals and populations [6]. A QI intervention may be also described as a systems-level strategy aimed at reducing a quality gap (the difference between health care processes or outcomes observed in practice and those potentially attainable based on evidence-based knowledge) for a group of patients representative of those cared for in routine clinical practice. Different categories of QI interventions described in the Closing the Gap series are listed in Table 2.1. Once an intervention is selected, different analytic tools may be used to monitor improvement over time. Specific tools include control charts, fishbone diagrams, histograms, Pareto charts, run charts, and scatter diagrams [7]. A measurement strategy should include a diverse array of measures—clinical quality, practice transformation, provider and staff satisfaction, patient experience, and efficiency [6].

It is possible that this comprehensive approach could be adapted to narrow a health or health care gap if implemented in a targeted way (i.e., institutions that treat predominantly minority populations as well as organizations that care for patients from a wide variety of subgroups) or if they could impact disparities at the population level [2]. For those invested in eliminating disparities, QI offers a dynamic platform by which to address modifiable care delivery variables, instead of attempting to ameliorate less readily modifiable factors such as poverty, crime, and implicit bias among clinical care providers [8–10]. QI also has the potential to address disparities by employing a sequential and iterative process targeting various aspects of care delivery. QI initiatives may impact health disparities by facilitating change at any of four levels: the experience of the patients, the performance of microsystems of care (i.e., individual health care providers and teams), the functioning of health care organizations, and the operation of the health care environment [6, 11].

The connection between disparities and QI has been promoted by several federal agencies in their initiatives to address disparities. In its 2001 report *Crossing the Quality Chasm*, the Institute of Medicine (IOM) recommended that health care be

Table 2.1 Commonly used quality improvement strategies

QI strategy	Examples
Patient education	• Classes • Parent and family education • Patient pamphlets • Intensive education strategies promoting self-management of chronic conditions
Promotion of self-management	• Postcards or calls to patients
Patient reminder systems	• Materials and devices promoting self-management
Provider education	• Workshops and conferences • Educational outreach visits (e.g., academic detailing) • Distribution of educational materials
Provider reminder systems	• Reminders in charts for providers • Computer-based reminders for providers • Computer-based decision support
Facilitated relay of clinical data to providers	• Transmission of clinical data from outpatient specialty clinic to primary care provider by means other than medical record (e.g., phone call or fax)
Audit and feedback	• Feedback of performance to individual providers • Quality indicators and reports • National/state quality report cards • Publicly released performance data • Benchmarking—provision of outcomes data from top performers for comparison with provider's own data
Organizational change	• Case management, disease management • Total Quality Management, Cycles of Quality Improvement • Multidisciplinary teams • Change from paper to computer-based records • Increased staffing • Skill mix changes
Other	• Guideline adherence • Care manager • Collaborative care model

safe, efficient, effective, timely, patient-centered, and equitable [6]. Health equity was subsequently elevated to a cross-cutting domain that should be considered within and across each of the other domains. The Agency for Healthcare Research and Quality (AHRQ) has codified the important link between quality and health disparities with its annual quality and disparity reports [12]. Legislation has also promoted this connection. The Affordable Care Act of 2010 required improved collection of race/ethnicity data and reporting of quality performance measures stratified according to race/ethnicity. The combination of these federal efforts and regulatory policy changes have provided further impetus to incorporate QI as a core strategy to address modifiable aspects of care delivery that largely contribute to disparities [13, 14].

Evidence Base for Disparities-Focused QI Interventions

As described by Weinick and Hasnan-Wynia [15], the anticipated outcomes of successful QI initiatives may follow three specific trajectories, all with distinct impact on disparities. The most ideal path would occur when a QI intervention results in disparity reduction or elimination. In this instance, the QI intervention would improve care for all children but have an amplified and heightened effect on the care of underserved children experiencing disparities. In a second path, a QI intervention may improve quality at the same rate for all groups. In such a scenario, if implementation of an intervention improves quality equally for all groups, disparities remain constant. Multiple studies from the adult literature have documented that disparities persist after implementation of overall successful QI interventions [16–19]. In a third trajectory, a QI intervention may result in differential rates of uptake or effect of an evidence-based intervention. If the benefit of a QI intervention relies on individual patient responses or access to care, individuals with access to greater resources, social networks, or social capital may be better positioned to experience benefits of the program. In these situations, disadvantaged children may benefit less, with a consequential widening of gaps in care between groups. If a provider or health system in a high-minority area lacks the resources to implement a particular QI intervention (e.g., decision support tool) that is implemented elsewhere, the gap between well-resourced practices and poorly resourced practices may widen. Additionally, QI interventions with demonstrated efficacy in majority populations may lead to initiatives that have efficacy only in those groups, further widening disparities. Lastly, QI interventions that involve provider profiling may penalize physicians who care for underserved children who are relatively sicker, poorer, or non-English speaking [20]. Such interventions may, in turn, unintentionally incentivize physicians to select away from such challenging patient subgroups. The phenomenon of QI interventions exacerbating disparities has been demonstrated in the adult QI literature. In one study, the public release of coronary artery bypass grafting report cards in New York was associated with a widening of the disparity in grafting use between white and racial/ethnic minority populations [21]. The study highlighted the potential unintended consequences of public reporting—physician avoidance of high-risk patients to improve their individual quality ratings.

Several reviews have explored the evidence base for QI interventions as effective strategies to reduce health disparities. A systematic review by Beach et al. summarized controlled trials of interventions targeted at health care providers to improve health care quality or reduce disparities in care for racial/ethnic minorities [22]. Twenty-seven studies met criteria for review. Almost all (n = 26) took place in the primary care setting, and most (n = 19) centered on improving provision of preventive services. QI interventions tested included tracking/reminders, provider education, bypass of physician, structured patient questionnaire, remote simultaneous translation, subspecialty consult, and defibrillators on emergency vehicles. A number interventions were multi-faceted (n = 9). Only three studies targeted pediatricians. Overall, the systematic review concluded that there was little evidence to support the use of QI interventions to specifically reduce disparities. A subsequent review by McPheeters et al. attempted to identify evidence about the effectiveness of QI strategies to reduce disparities and determine whether there are harms related to QI interventions focused on disparities [23]. This review sought studies that described a QI intervention and measured potential changes in the inequity of care between patient groups with pre-specified clinical conditions. No pediatric studies met inclusion criteria. The review, consisting of 14 studies, concluded there was insufficient evidence to demonstrate the effectiveness of QI interventions to address disparity gaps. The authors of the report summarized methodological challenges to synthesis and interpretation in conducting such a review. These included heterogeneity in the study populations, target clinical conditions, and interventions. Other difficulties cited included a paucity of studies assessing gaps between groups and inconsistencies in how QI studies are indexed in the medical literature.

Challenges to Using QI to Address Disparities

QI strategies encounter various challenges and unintended consequences to reducing inequities in care [20]. Several challenges exist in methodology. Many health care institutions do not systematically or routinely collect data on race/ethnicity, primary language, preferred language for care, sexual orientation, or geographical residence (urban, suburban, rural). Consequently, data according to relevant subgroups may not be available at the time that QI interventions are chosen, implemented, monitored, and evaluated. Another difficulty in assessing the impact of any health care intervention on disparities is that research must demonstrate effectiveness across multiple planes. Effectiveness must be shown using a non-intervention comparison group, and simultaneously, a disparity in outcome must be narrowed in the intervention group, but not in the control group. Consequently, for a QI intervention to be effective, both intervention effectiveness and disparity reduction effectiveness must be demonstrated [2]. The intervention must be more effective for the disadvantaged group than for advantaged groups. Therefore, effectiveness cannot be determined when the intervention is only targeted at disadvantaged individuals or groups. While such work has the potential to provide great insights, research that simultaneously demonstrates effectiveness in changing outcomes and reducing disparities between two or more groups is substantially complex and therefore rare.

Challenges also occur with respect to patients and providers [20]. These challenges take place at multiple levels, from the specific patient population to the health care system. For patients, there are several potential barriers. First, target populations in underserved communities may not have the capacity or time to fully engage in QI interventions due to systemic barriers including economic, health literacy, cultural, or language factors as well as competing priorities. Second, individual patient preferences regarding care delivery may not be routinely incorporated into quality improvement performance measures. Previous studies have demonstrated that patients may not comply with specific types of screenings due to individual preference [24]. If the design of performance measures does not take into account patient perspectives and preferences, potential consequences include decreased patient satisfaction and provider satisfaction [20]. Third, public reporting interventions may provide information to patients which may negatively influence patient-provider relationships, particularly when patients have limited ability to change providers due to geographic or insurance restrictions [20, 25, 26]. It may be difficult to repair relationships when trust has been lost with hospitals or individual practitioners.

Disparities-focused QI interventions also carry risks for clinical providers. QI directed focus on a particular topic may displace counseling for other topics during patient encounters [20]. In well child care, such topics may include child development, sleep hygiene, injury prevention, and obesity prevention. If the intervention focuses on a specific aspect of a general topic (e.g., obesity), other aspects of that topic may be neglected. For example, an obesity QI intervention focused on physical activity may take away from discussion on nutrition. There is also concern for physician "measurement fixation", a phenomenon in which the provider becomes predominantly focused on improving rates on specified measures rather than improving patient outcomes overall [20]. For example, a QI intervention focused on asthma may lead to a high rate of inhaled corticosteroid initiation, even in cases where not indicated. QI strategies such as pay-for-performance programs and public reporting have the potential to undermine care for underserved populations in multiple ways. These include incentivizing clinical providers to avoid caring for children who are perceived to be high-risk and financially penalizing providers without the requisite resources to participate in costly QI programs. There is also concern that such interventions may negatively influence perception of providers in resource poor settings. If publicly released reports reveal that such providers do poorly on certain quality metrics, patients may feel less confidence in their providers or seek care elsewhere. Underlying issues of mistrust with the medical community may be exacerbated. Concurrently, providers who don't have the resources to successfully achieve QI benchmarks may become discouraged and leave underserved neighborhoods for employment in more highly resourced settings. These set of circumstances may create a situation with fewer providers available to care for an underserved and socially complex pediatric population.

Future of QI in Addressing Pediatric Health Disparities

Despite an evolving evidence base still in a nascent stage and substantial, multi-level barriers to conducting QI interventions in underserved communities, QI continues to represent a promising platform for addressing the modifiable components of health care delivery that cause and propagate disparities. As researchers and policy makers have noted, the difficulty in establishing a disparities-based QI agenda is the multifactorial nature of disparities attributable to the social determinants of health. In order to overcome these challenges, fundamental paradigm shifts must occur in how both health disparities research and QI interventions have been historically conducted. Outlined below are five key areas of focus for clinicians, researchers, and policy makers invested in exploring the potential of QI to address health disparities [27].

Consideration of Comparators

Historically, interventions directed at reducing disparities require data on both minority or underserved group in question and the majority group being used as a standard population. This approach allows the disparity between the two groups to be tracked and monitored over time. While health disparities research has traditionally relied on such comparators, such an approach in QI evaluations may require reconsideration for several reasons. First, as already discussed, baseline data on demographic variables (e.g., race/ethnicity, primary language, sexual orientation, geographic place of residence) are not routinely available for QI interventions given variable and inconsistent collection practices in clinical settings. While legislation and professional organizations have endorsed more rigorous collection of demographic data, such practices have not been widely adopted due to limited standardization in collection processes, resources, infrastructure, and appropriate incentives or penalties to encourage meaningful commitment and participation. Second, there are no standards or benchmarks for what constitutes a clinically relevant disparity or disparity reduction. Third, QI studies may be underpowered to detect statistically significant differences due to insufficient numbers of children in relevant subgroups. Fourth, since many providers who serve vulnerable populations tend to serve predominantly minority patients, non-minority reference groups may not be readily available within the same clinical setting.

Given these unique aspects of disparities research, QI strategies to address disparities must accordingly take new approaches. Some QI studies may be best conducted by targeting well-documented, high risk subgroups of children for intervention rather than trying to assess solutions for all children of varying backgrounds simultaneously in a single clinical setting. This approach will facilitate customization and cultural tailoring of QI interventions, whereby specific root causes of disparities can be targeted, either initially in intervention design or iteratively over time in response to data analysis. Such an approach may also heighten the efficiency and effectiveness of interventions. An increasing number of QI interventions are using this strategy to improve care for underserved children [28–30]. Comparison of outcomes according to relevant subgroups will still be critical to monitor progress and mitigate against exacerbation of disparities with QI initiatives. However, for customized interventions targeted towards a single, high-risk subgroup of children, such comparisons will not be feasible. Alternatively, comparisons made within a specifically targeted subgroup, ideally between care settings serving similar populations, should be considered for robustly evaluating the impact of QI interventions.

Rigor of QI Interventions Addressing Disparities

Methodological rigor in the development, implementation, and evaluation of QI interventions represents a major priority for levering QI strategies to reduce disparities. Uncontrolled, observational study designs used historically by some QI interventions impede the ability to understand what works [27, 31, 32]. This is especially important for low-resource health care delivery settings, which are less likely to have available a QI team of their own developing internal interventions, and more likely to be reliant on approaches designed and implemented at well-resourced institutions. Improved methodological rigor and reporting from studies at well-resourced settings will help those with fewer resources identify strategies that are more likely to work in various settings.

Investigators undertaking QI should utilize a diverse array of rigorous methods and analyses including stepped wedge design, interrupted time series analysis, and statistical process control [33–35]. These approaches are especially critical for disparities-focused interventions because they assess effectiveness in real-world settings, with attention to influence of structural and subconscious processes that contribute to disparities but pose challenges in measurement. They also differentiate intervention effect from temporal and contextual factors. This is essential for successful translation of interventions from one setting to another. Furthermore, wherever possible, real time data should be stratified according to relevant subgroups (e.g., race/ethnicity, language).

Understanding Context and Intended Mechanism of Intervention

In selecting and evaluating interventions, disparities-focused QI interventions would also benefit from careful consideration of intervention mechanism and context. To understand the likely impact of a QI intervention, researchers who seek evidence-based strategies from the literature or other institutions should consider the care structure, processes, and outcomes in the targeted health care setting; the context surrounding those care delivery attributes; how those compare with the ones described in previous works; and whether they vary for different groups of patients. For example, family-centered rounds have been widely implemented in inpatient settings, providing a new approach to engage families and improve communication [36, 37]. However, the specific aspects of engaging and communicating with families with limited English proficiency were not considered or accounted

for in seminal studies of family-centered rounds. Even when professional inter-
preters were incorporated into family-centered rounds, the communication and
overall experience for families with limited English proficiency differed from
those proficient in English. These differences highlight the challenges inherent to
implementing a single QI intervention across multiple groups that have different
preexisting processes. Researchers increasingly recognize that many low-income
and racial/ethnic minority families interface with the health care system in ways
that fundamentally differ from other groups. A study by Patterson et al. reported on
a QI intervention developed to facilitate provision of overdue well-child services
such as immunizations, developmental screening, and anticipatory guidance at
urgent care visits [38]. The intervention was developed for families that potentially
face logistical and financial barriers in regularly attending routine well child care
visits. These studies from the literature highlight the importance of understanding
the anticipated mechanisms of action of the intervention and potential barriers or
facilitators to uptake or effectiveness. In order to enhance the effectiveness of an
intervention developed among other populations, it may be important to incorporate novel, low-cost delivery approaches with high utilization rates among vulnerable populations. For example, text messaging has been used as a strategy to
improve medication adherence for chronic conditions such as HIV, sickle cell disease, and diabetes. Careful attention should also be paid attention to the context in
which an intervention is conducted, including the available resources, organiza-
tional structure, leadership commitment, and data infrastructure [39]. All of these
considerations are critical in ensuring effective translation from one setting or
population to another.

Incorporating the Social Determinants of Health

Direct engagement of the social determinants of health in QI interventions has the
potential to simultaneously improve care in health care settings and more broadly
advance population health in communities. It is a unique opportunity to assess the
impact of influences such as income, education, housing, and other environmental
factors on health maintenance, health care utilization, and ultimately health outcomes. Increasingly, researchers are incorporating community factors into QI
interventions in order to improve community health at multiple levels, beyond
those typically addressed in health care access or service delivery. A study by Beck
et al. addressing pediatric asthma used a geographic social risk index to predict
asthma-related reutilization [40]. Such geographic data could also be used to
inform community-level preventive approaches, targeting neighborhood hot spots
that would benefit from public health initiatives. In a study by Woods et al., investigators developed and tested a QI intervention for pediatric asthma using community-based participatory research [30]. The intervention addressed multiple social
determinants of health, including exposure to asthma triggers found in poor housing and school buildings and chronic stress due to community violence. Intervention

components consisted of high efficiency particulate air vacuums, bedding encasements, and extermination as needed. Community health workers provided culturally competent education about asthma management and addressed personal beliefs about asthma.

Leveraging Community Resources

Many of the vulnerable populations who could benefit from QI interventions tend to receive care and/or live in resource poor settings. Consequently, promotion of QI in these areas may require significant modification and adaption of existing interventions, careful attention to financial and intellectual resources, and novel approaches to funding and implementation. Prior research on health disparities collaboratives in community health centers demonstrates that QI initiatives focused on underserved populations can be effective with appropriate funding [41]. Without adequate funding, investigators must develop meaningful collaborations with community-based organizations in order to leverage available community assets and increase the sustainability of initiatives. As an example, use of community health workers has been shown to improve health outcomes for children with chronic conditions by establishing links between clinic and community members through education and coaching [42]. Such collaboration and integration into ongoing community programs may facilitate development of QI interventions more likely to meet the needs of communities. These community partnerships may also lead to funding opportunities through agencies such as the Patient Centered Outcomes Research Institute (PCORI), where patient and stakeholder engagement is a core requirement for research funding. PCORI, which has an Addressing Disparities Study Panel, requires applicants to actively incorporate patients and relevant stakeholders in helping to identify key research questions, select study designs, choose comparators and outcomes, identify and recruit study participants, develop research materials, and interpret and disseminate findings.

Conclusions

With health care quality and equity established as central tenets in continuous health care system redesign, rigorously conducted QI interventions represent a core strategy towards achieving the triple aim of enhancing patient experience, lowering costs, and improving population health [43]. For underserved children, QI has the potential to address historic inequities in health care delivery. The medical literature has yet to demonstrate widespread benefit of QI interventions in ameliorating or eliminating disparities. However, the lack of findings may speak to the complex nature of health disparities, study design and evaluation challenges, structural barriers inherent in underserved communities, and the paucity of disparities focused

QI research in child health. Successful integration of QI and health disparities research will require novel approaches to identifying comparators; improved methodological rigor in selecting and evaluating interventions; heightened consideration of context; increased attention to social determinants of health; and leveraging of community assets. More practically, QI researchers must develop collaborative partnerships with frontline clinical providers and community leaders committed to improving the care of underserved children. Such initiatives may foster more tailored, efficient interventions and inform programs to improve clinical outcomes, and ultimately community and population health.

References

1. Flores G, Committee On Pediatric R. Technical report – racial and ethnic disparities in the health and health care of children. Pediatrics. 2010;125:e979–e1020.
2. McPheeters ML, Kripalani S, Peterson NB, et al. Closing the quality gap: revisiting the state of the science (vol. 3: quality improvement interventions to address health disparities). Evidence report/technology assessment. 2012:1–475.
3. Donabedian A. The effectiveness of quality assurance. Int J Qual Health Care. 1996;8:401–7.
4. A critical analysis of quality improvement strategies: closing the gap. Agency for Healthcare Research and Quality, Rockville, MD. 2004. At http://www.ahrq.gov/research/findings/factsheets/quality/qgapfact/index.html. Accessed 5 July 2018.
5. Baily M, Bottrell M, Lynn J, Jennings B. The ethics of using QI methods to improve health care quality and safety. Hasting Cent Rep. 2006;36:S1–S40.
6. Institute of Medicine. Crossing the quality chasm: a new health system for the 21st century. Washington, D.C.: National Academies Press; 2001.
7. Safety net medical home initiative, Altman Dautoff D, Van Borkulo N, Daniel D. Quality improvement strategy: tools to make and measure improvement. In: Phillips KE, Weir V, editors. Safety net medical home initiative implementation guide series. 2nd ed. Seattle, WA: Qualis Health and The MacColl Center for Health Care Innovation at the Group Health Research Institute; 2013.
8. Katz AL, Webb SA, Committee On B. Informed consent in decision-making in pediatric practice. Pediatrics. 2016;138:e20161485.
9. Consequences of growing up poor. New York: Russell Sage Foundation; 1997.
10. Green AR, Carney DR, Pallin DJ, et al. Implicit bias among physicians and its prediction of thrombolysis decisions for black and white patients. J Gen Intern Med. 2007;22:1231–8.
11. Berwick DM. A user's manual for the IOM's 'Quality Chasm' report. Health Aff. 2002;21:80–90.
12. National healthcare quality and disparities reports.
13. Beal AC. High-quality health care: the essential route to eliminating disparities and achieving health equity. Health Aff. 2011;30:1868–71.
14. Beal AC, Hasnain-Wynia R. Disparities and quality: the next phase for high-performing pediatric care. Acad Pediatr. 2013;13:S21–2.
15. Weinick RM, Hasnain-Wynia R. Quality improvement efforts under health reform: how to ensure that they help reduce disparities – not increase them. Health Aff. 2011;30:1837–43.
16. Arean PA, Ayalon L, Hunkeler E, et al. Improving depression care for older, minority patients in primary care. Med Care. 2005;43:381–90.
17. Sequist TD, Adams A, Zhang F, Ross-Degnan D, Ayanian JZ. Effect of quality improvement on racial disparities in diabetes care. Arch Intern Med. 2006;166:675–81.

18. Trivedi AN, Zaslavsky AM, Schneider EC, Ayanian JZ. Trends in the quality of care and racial disparities in Medicare managed care. New Engl J Med. 2005;353:692–700.
19. Trivedi AN, Grebla RC, Wright SM, Washington DL. Despite improved quality of care in the Veterans Affairs health system, racial disparity persists for important clinical outcomes. Health Aff. 2011;30:707–15.
20. Bardach NS, Cabana MD. The unintended consequences of quality improvement. Curr Opin Pediatr. 2009;21:777–82.
21. Werner RM, Asch DA, Polsky D. Racial profiling: the unintended consequences of coronary artery bypass graft report cards. Circulation. 2005;111:1257–63.
22. Beach MC, Gary TL, Price EG, et al. Improving health care quality for racial/ethnic minorities: a systematic review of the best evidence regarding provider and organization interventions. BMC Public Health. 2006;6:104.
23. McPheeters ML, Kripalani S, Peterson NB, et al. Quality improvement interventions to address health disparities. Closing the quality gap: revisiting the state of the science. Rockville, MD: Agency for Healthcare Research and Quality; 2012. AHRQ Publication 12-E009-EF. Evidence Report 208.
24. Walter LC, Davidowitz NP, Heineken PA, Covinsky KE. Pitfalls of converting practice guidelines into quality measures: lessons learned from a VA performance measure. JAMA. 2004;291:2466–70.
25. Britto MT, DeVellis RF, Hornung RW, DeFriese GH, Atherton HD, Slap GB. Health care preferences and priorities of adolescents with chronic illnesses. Pediatrics. 2004;114:1272–80.
26. Faber M, Bosch M, Wollersheim H, Leatherman S, Grol R. Public reporting in health care: how do consumers use quality-of-care information? A systematic review. Med Care. 2009;47:1–8.
27. Lion KC, Raphael JL. Partnering health disparities research with quality improvement science in pediatrics. Pediatrics. 2015;135:354–61.
28. Chin MH, Alexander-Young M, Burnet DL. Health care quality-improvement approaches to reducing child health disparities. Pediatrics. 2009;124(Suppl 3):S224–36.
29. Lob SH, Boer JH, Porter PG, Nunez D, Fox P. Promoting best-care practices in childhood asthma: quality improvement in community health centers. Pediatrics. 2011;128:20–8.
30. Woods ER, Bhaumik U, Sommer SJ, et al. Community asthma initiative: evaluation of a quality improvement program for comprehensive asthma care. Pediatrics. 2012;129:465–72.
31. McDonald KM, Schultz EM, Chang C. Evaluating the state of quality-improvement science through evidence synthesis: insights from the closing the quality gap series. Perm J. 2013;17:52–61.
32. Rotter T, Kinsman L, James E, Machotta A, Steyerberg EW. The quality of the evidence base for clinical pathway effectiveness: room for improvement in the design of evaluation trials. BMC Med Res Methodol. 2012;12:80.
33. Wagner AK, Soumerai SB, Zhang F, Ross-Degnan D. Segmented regression analysis of interrupted time series studies in medication use research. J Clin Pharm Ther. 2002;27:299–309.
34. Benneyan JC, Lloyd RC, Plsek PE. Statistical process control as a tool for research and healthcare improvement. Qual Saf Health Care. 2003;12:458–64.
35. Brown CA, Lilford RJ. The stepped wedge trial design: a systematic review. BMC Med Res Methodol. 2006;6:54.
36. Mittal VS, Sigrest T, Ottolini MC, et al. Family-centered rounds on pediatric wards: a PRIS network survey of US and Canadian hospitalists. Pediatrics. 2010;126:37–43.
37. Kuo DZ, Sisterhen LL, Sigrest TE, Biazo JM, Aitken ME, Smith CE. Family experiences and pediatric health services use associated with family-centered rounds. Pediatrics. 2012;130:299–305.
38. Patterson BL, Gregg WM, Biggers C, Barkin S. Improving delivery of EPSDT well-child care at acute visits in an academic pediatric practice. Pediatrics. 2012;130:e988–95.
39. Kaplan HC, Brady PW, Dritz MC, et al. The influence of context on quality improvement success in health care: a systematic review of the literature. Milbank Q. 2010;88:500–59.

40. Beck AF, Simmons JM, Huang B, Kahn RS. Geomedicine: area-based socioeconomic measures for assessing risk of hospital reutilization among children admitted for asthma. Am J Public Health. 2012;102:2308–14.
41. Chin MH. Quality improvement implementation and disparities: the case of the health disparities collaboratives. Med Care. 2010;48:668–75.
42. Raphael JL, Rueda A, Lion KC, Giordano TP. The role of lay health workers in pediatric chronic disease: a systematic review. Acad Pediatr. 2013;13:408–20.
43. Berwick DM, Nolan TW, Whittington J. The triple aim: care, health, and cost. Health Aff. 2008;27:759–69.

Chapter 3
Community Health Worker Interventions

Michelle A. Lopez

Interventions involving community health workers (CHWs) are another mechanism to engage vulnerable patient populations and address healthcare disparities. As defined by the American Public Health Association in 2009, CHWs are "frontline public health workers who are trusted members of and/or have an unusually close understanding of the community served" and, as such, CHWs are able to "serve as a liaison, link, or intermediary between health/social services and the community to facilitate access to services and improve the quality and cultural competence of service delivery" [1]. While other definitions of CHWs exist under the United States Department of Labor, Department of State Health Services, Patient Protection and Affordable Care Act and Health Resources and Services Administration, common elements include a special connection to a community and a purpose of improving access to care and promoting health equity [2]. CHWs are also referred to by several other names including lay health workers, community care coordinators, community health educators, outreach workers, peer educator, promotores de salud (health promoters), and patient navigators [2]. Many of the terms are used interchangeably. However, in some cases, the exact terminology refers to specific roles. For example, patient navigator duties fall under a subset of CHW responsibilities, and patient navigation services can be CHWs, nurses, or social workers. Patient navigators are often assigned to specific patients for a particular purpose [2].

CHWs serve as vital team members in addressing health disparities. While there are complex interactions of determinants leading to health disparities, CHWs are often equipped to address several of the contributing factors. Because of their relationships with communities and demographic backgrounds, CHWs can develop rapport with racially and ethnically diverse communities who may otherwise be

M. A. Lopez (✉)
Pediatrics-Hospital Medicine, Baylor College of Medicine, Houston, TX, USA

© The Author(s), under exclusive licence to Springer Nature Switzerland AG 2018
M. A. Lopez et al., *Disparities in Child Health*, SpringerBriefs in Public Health,
https://doi.org/10.1007/978-3-030-03210-4_3

mistrusting of medical professionals. CHWs who speak the language, know the customs, and are aware of barriers, can provide care that is tailored to the culture of the participants. As such, CHWs are better equipped to work through patients' concerns and potentially help change behaviors. Additionally, they are able to build partnerships with the community organizations and help patients access needed resources. Overall, it is also more feasible to reach rural communities with CHWs than social workers because of job force supply.

In particular, CHWs are often well equipped to help address health disparities in the pediatric population. Social determinants of health are known to impact children's health and well-being, and patients living in poverty are especially vulnerable to these effects [3]. As CHWs are able to work one-on-one at the family level, they can address the child's healthcare needs in the context of the family social and economic needs. With expertise in navigating the healthcare system and resources, CHWs can connect families to programs such as Medicaid transport services to get to medical appointments or sliding scale clinics and pharmacies for those who are uninsured. CHWs can also help families navigate complex application and renewal processes for public insurance. For children with chronic conditions, CHWs can help families engage the school system and obtain in school therapy services and accommodations for disabilities. CHWs are also in a position to respond to the changing needs of pediatric patients as they grow. Children with chronic conditions have evolving health demands, and eventually transition from pediatric to adult services, which can be a difficult process for families. CHWs working closely with specific populations and communities can be responsive to these dynamic changes and help patients through changes in healthcare settings.

The first description of a community health promoter exists from the 1950s/1960s [4], but CHWs have gained more attention from national organizations and in public policy over recent years. In 2009, the United States Department of Labor created a standard occupational classification for the field of CHWs, followed by listing it as an "apprenticeable" occupation in 2010 [5]. The Patient Protection and Affordable Care Act of 2010 provided opportunities to increase the role of CHWs in state Medicaid programs under preventative care services, chronic disease management and innovative cost savings plans [6]. Most recently, in 2013, Centers for Medicare and Medicaid Services (CMS) allowed for the potential reimbursement of preventive services provided by CHWs [5].

CHWs function in a multitude of roles. The core competencies of CHWs have been summarized as (1) bridging/cultural mediation between communities and the health care systems; (2) providing culturally appropriate and accessible health education and information; (3) assuring that people get the services they need; (4) providing informal counseling and social support; (5) advocating for individual and community needs; (6) providing direct services; and (7) building individual and community capacity [7].

Evidence supports the value of CHW-based interventions in multiple areas including preventive medicine and the management of chronic illnesses. CHWs have demonstrated a successful role in promoting vaccination uptake amongst young children. An intervention supported by community volunteers serving in the role of CHWs provided immunization outreach, vaccine tracking and phone follow up to parents of the children under 2 years of age in an ambulatory setting in New York [8]. This intervention demonstrated a 2.8 greater odds of the intervention group obtaining vaccines compared to the control [8]. In adult chronic disease management for Hispanic patients with Type II Diabetes and cardiovascular disease, CHW-based interventions resulted in a significant decrease in Hemoglobin A1C [9] as well as total cholesterol, low-density lipoprotein and weight control practices [10]. In pediatric asthma management, an intensive intervention involving CHWs demonstrated several significant benefits. Through a community-based participatory research project, CHWs functioned as "community environmental specialists (CESs)" [11]. They received training on behavior change, asthma environmental triggers, pest management, access to medical services, and community referral options [11]. The CESs were assigned to households of children 7–11 years old with persistent asthma symptoms and completed a minimum of nine home visits over 1 year [11]. The CES intervention was effective in improving patient lung function, reducing frequency of asthma symptoms, decreasing unscheduled medical visits, reducing caregiver reports of depressive symptoms, and improving household air quality [11]. The results of this study were highly encouraging and demonstrate the potential health benefits of robust CHW-based interventions in pediatric populations. Similarly, a systematic review of the role of CHWs in pediatric chronic disease found lay health worker interventions lead to modest improvements in reduced urgent care use, decreased symptoms, and improved parental psychosocial outcomes [12]. However, not all studies have been as successful. In one study to reduce tobacco smoke exposure in Latino children, trained CHWs completed six home and telephone sessions aimed at problem solving and found no difference in pre-intervention and post-intervention comparisons of nicotine exposure [13]. The level of training CHWs receive and the wide range of interactions between CHWs and study participants are limitations in generalizing outcomes and in the overall development of the field. As reported in a systematic review of CHW-based interventions, CHWs interacted with participants in an array of locations, with a spectrum of materials at various levels of intensity [14]. These factors in combination with a lack of reporting detail in many of the studies examined, make it difficult to generate guidelines on CHW-based interventions [14], and further high quality studies are needed. To maximize success, CHW interventions should be approached systematically, providing CHWs adequate training for the duties expected, and with sufficient oversight by experienced healthcare professionals.

Despite the heterogeneous nature of CHW training, roles, interventions and outcomes, studying the cost effectiveness of these programs is essential in order to continue to develop the field. In 2015, CHWs had a mean annual wage of $40,150 in 2015 which was less than professions who could provide comparable services including behavior disorder counselors ($42,920), clinical social workers ($54,020) and dietitians ($58,410) [15]. A systematic review of 19 economic evaluation studies aimed at improving child health outcomes with CHW-based interventions found all were either cost-effective or highly cost-effective based on their respective countries [16]. Cost-effective interventions in the United States included a program to increase exclusive breastfeeding in low-income women and demonstrated infants in the intervention group had fewer sick visits than infants in the usual care group [17]. CHW-based interventions to address health disparities have the potential to result in cost-savings.

Evidence-based recommendations for CHWs as a field are beginning to reach more of a consensus amongst multiple stakeholders. Key directions for the future are the development of a standardized core CHW curriculum, core competency CHW certification, provisions for supervision of CHWs by health care professionals, CMS reimbursement of medical practices for CHW services, and inclusion of CHWs in the development of certification requirements [18]. A national survey of CHWs found variations across the United States in current training practices ranging from formal classes to on-the-job training [19]. A minimum of five states including Massachusetts, Minnesota, Ohio, Oregon and Texas currently require CHW certification for practice or reimbursement, and other states are currently examining their regulations [20]. As national organizations and state regulations continue to recognize the potential roles of CHWs in advancing population health with cost-effective strategies, the field will continue to progress. Public health workers and researchers should remain aware of the demonstrated value of CHWs and their ability to address health disparities in targeted populations. In particular, CHWs are well equipped to address the unique needs of vulnerable pediatric patients and their families.

References

1. American Public Health Association. Support for community health workers to increase health access and to reduce health inequities. Policy Statement 20091. 2009.
2. Centers for Disease Control. Community health workers (CHWs) promoting policy and systems change to expand employment of community health workers (CHWs). https://www.cdc.gov/dhdsp/chw_elearning/index.html. Accessed 10 Sept 2017.
3. Chung EK, Siegel BS, Garg A, et al. Screening for social determinants of health among children and families living in poverty: a guide for clinicians. Curr Probl Pediatr Adolesc Health Care. 2016;46:135–53.
4. Lehman U, Sanders D. Community health workers: what do we know about them? The state of the evidence on programmes, activities, costs and impact on health outcomes of using community health workers. Geneva: World Health Organization; 2007.
5. American Public Health Association. Support for community health worker leadership in determining workforce standards for training and credentialing. Policy Statement 201414. 2014.
6. Katzen A, Morgan M. Affordable care act opportunities for community health workers. How Medicaid preventive services, Medicaid health homes, and state innovation models are including community health workers. Harvard Center for Health Law and Policy Innovation. 2014.
7. Rosenthal EL, Wiggins N, Ingram M, Mayfield-Johnson S, De Zapien JG. Community health workers then and now: an overview of national studies aimed at defining the field. J Ambul Care Manage. 2011;34:247–59.

8. Barnes K, Friedman SM, Brickner Namerow P, Honig J. Impact of community volunteers on immunization rates of children younger than 2 years. Arch Pediatr Adolesc Med. 1999;153:518–24.
9. Prezio EA, Cheng D, Balasubramanian BA, Shuval K, Kendzor DE, Culica D. Community diabetes education (CoDE) for uninsured Mexican Americans: a randomized controlled trial of a culturally tailored diabetes education and management program led by a community health worker. Diabetes Res Clin Pract. 2013;100:19–28.
10. Balcazar HG, de Heer H, Rosenthal L, et al. A promotores de salud intervention to reduce cardiovascular disease risk in a high-risk Hispanic border population, 2005–2008. Prev Chronic Dis. 2010;7:A28.
11. Parker EA, Israel BA, Robins TG, et al. Evaluation of community action against asthma: a community health worker intervention to improve children's asthma-related health by reducing household environmental triggers for asthma. Health Educ Behav. 2008;35:376–95.
12. Raphael JL, Rueda A, Lion KC, Giordano TP. The role of lay health workers in pediatric chronic disease: a systematic review. Acad Pediatr. 2013;13:408–20.
13. Conway TL, Woodruff SI, Edwards CC, Hovell MF, Klein J. Intervention to reduce environmental tobacco smoke exposure in Latino children: null effects on hair biomarkers and parent reports. Tob Control. 2004;13:90–2.
14. Viswanathan MKJ, Nishikawa B, Morgan LC, Thieda P, Honeycutt A, Lohr KN, Jonas D. Outcomes of community health worker interventions. Evidence report/technology assessment No. 181 (Prepared by the RTI International–University of North Carolina Evidence-based Practice Center under Contract No. 290 2007 10056 I.) AHRQ publication No. 09-E014. Rockville, MD: Agency for Healthcare Research and Quality. 2009.
15. Community Health Worker Salary. US news and world report. https://money.usnews.com/careers/best-jobs/community-health-worker/salary. Accessed 22 Nov 2017.
16. Nkonki L, Tugendhaft A, Hofman K. A systematic review of economic evaluations of CHW interventions aimed at improving child health outcomes. Hum Resour Health. 2017;15:19.
17. Pugh LC, Milligan RA, Frick KD, Spatz D, Bronner Y. Breastfeeding duration, costs, and benefits of a support program for low-income breastfeeding women. Birth. 2002;29:95–100.
18. National Center for Chronic Disease Prevention and Health Promotion. Policy evidence assessment report: community health worker policy components. https://www.cdc.gov/dhdsp/pubs/docs/chw_evidence_assessment_report.pdf. Accessed 10 Sept 2017.
19. Kash BA, May ML, Tai-Seale M. Community health worker training and certification programs in the United States: findings from a national survey. Health Policy. 2007;80:32–42.
20. Miller PBT, Katzen A. Community health worker credentialing state approaches. Harvard Center for Health Law and Policy Innovation. 2014.

Chapter 4
Technology-Based Interventions to Address Pediatric Health Disparities

Michelle A. Lopez

As we delve into interventions, it is important to consider that strategies aimed at improving disparate health outcomes may potentially have higher uptake and greater results in populations with better baseline health. The most successful strategies avoid widening disparities in their design. This section will explore potential benefits and barriers to Technology-Based Interventions.

Technology-Based Interventions

Technology-based interventions are one method to enhance patient engagement. Historically, concerns existed about the potential worsening of healthcare disparities in resource-limited populations. Data from the United States Department of Commerce in a report entitled *Falling Through the Net: Toward Digital Inclusion,* demonstrated racial and ethnic differences in the use of the Internet. Blacks and Hispanics Internet access was approximately half that of Whites in 2000 [1]. However, this gap has closed overtime. In a 2010 survey by the US Census Bureau, slightly over 50% of Black and Hispanics had access to internet in the home compared to 71% of homes overall [2] and data from the Pew Research Center in 2016, demonstrated internet use at 85–88% across all white, black and Hispanic groups and internet use at 88% of adults overall [3].

Computers, handheld devices, and cellular phones are occupying an increasing share of child activities. Between 2005 and 2010, children increased their use of media from all sources from 6.5 to 7.5 h/day [4]. Through media multi-tasking,

M. A. Lopez (✉)
Pediatrics-Hospital Medicine, Baylor College of Medicine, Houston, TX, USA

© The Author(s), under exclusive licence to Springer Nature Switzerland AG 2018   31
M. A. Lopez et al., *Disparities in Child Health*, SpringerBriefs in Public Health,
https://doi.org/10.1007/978-3-030-03210-4_4

Table 4.1 Healthy people 2020 health communication and health information technology impact on health, health care, and health equity

• Supporting shared decision-making between patients and providers
• Providing personalized self-management tools and resources
• Building social support networks
• Delivering accurate, accessible, and actionable health information that is targeted or tailored
• Facilitating the meaningful use of health IT and the exchange of health information among health care and public health professionals
• Enabling quick and informed responses to health risks and public health emergencies
• Increasing health literacy skills
• Providing new opportunities to connect with culturally diverse and hard-to-reach populations
• Providing sound principles in the design of programs and interventions that result in healthier behaviors

children may effectively consume an additional three hours of media content per week. Recent data reveals that 92% of adolescents report going online daily and approximately one-quarter reveal they are online constantly [5]. Evidence also demonstrates that technology use is high among adolescents with chronic conditions, including those from racial/ethnic minority backgrounds [6, 7].

The effects of internet-based interventions can be far reaching. As highlighted by Healthy People 2020 in Table 4.1, these include providing self-management tools and resources to patients, building social support networks, and connecting to culturally diverse and hard-to-reach populations. Examples of disadvantaged populations benefiting from technology-based strategies will be further explored below.

With the large majority of adults in the United States now having access to the Internet, strategies dependent on technology have the potential to reach a significant proportion of the population, even those from disadvantaged backgrounds. Furthermore, many adults use their phones to access the internet. Overall, 92% of US adults were estimated to have a cell phone in 2016 including 86% of individuals with household incomes less than $30,000 and 86% of individuals without a high school diploma or GED [3]. Thus, interventions involving use of smart phones are particularly promising in promoting health equity.

This use of mobile computing and communication technologies such as smart phones and wearable devices for health services and information is referred to as mHealth [8]. Systematic reviews examining the impact of mHealth demonstrate higher adherence with preventative care [9], increased self-management in Chronic Obstructive Pulmonary Disease [10] and improved glycemic control in Type II Diabetes [11]. A meta-analysis of mobile technology interventions for weight-loss found participants in text messaging based intervention programs had significantly greater weight loss than control patients [8]. In particular, multi-modal methodology reinforced positive behaviors. For example, one of the weight loss studies examined demonstrated significantly improved weight loss with the addition of texting and personalized feedback to an already successful social media and self-monitoring intervention [8]. For most conditions, long term follow up data is lacking and there is a paucity of evidence demonstrating cost-effective improvements in health outcomes. Key components of mHealth programs include a structured program with qualified interventionalist, patient self-monitoring, feedback and communication, social support and individualized tailoring [12]. When considering these interventions in disadvantaged populations, customization should consider age-related needs, language translation, culturally effective content, potential barriers to adherence based on access to recommended interventions.

As the healthcare community, public health workers and researchers consider targeted mHealth interventions, the potential benefits in the pediatric population are especially promising in preventative care and chronic disease management. Text message reminders can promote medical adherence and vaccination uptake. Appointment reminders via text resulted in a 14% decrease in no-show rates for pediatric appointments in a predominantly African American setting [13]. Additionally, in a study of urban, low-income families, children 11–18 years old whose parents who received a text message reminder for their meningococcal and tetanus–diphtheria–acellular pertussis immunizations were over twice as likely to be vaccinated [14]. Similarly, technology-based interventions have significant potential in pediatric chronic disease management, particularly when tailored to the targeted population. A study of adolescents and young adults with sickle cell disease found a prototype mobile app co-designed by their peers to be highly feasible and beneficial for disease management [7]. In chronic disease, technology is also changing traditional management practices and making compliance more feasible. In children with Type I Diabetes, continuous glucose monitoring (CGM) systems uses a small sensor wire inserted below the skin's surface [15]. This sensor provides measures of continuous glucose levels, which can be accessed by a using a mobile reader above the sensor wire [15]. These results can also be transmitted to parents via a cell phone app. This technology promotes adherence by alleviating the need for uncomfortable finger sticks and allows parents to monitor their child's glucose levels remotely. Unfortunately, CGM is costly and the system was only reimbursable by private insurances initially. As new mHealth technology becomes available, the medical community and policy makers must remain aware of inequities in availability for vulnerable populations, which have the potential to widen healthcare disparities.

Social media and social network sites are another way for technology to reach vulnerable populations. Social media brings social communities together regardless of geography, which allows for increased collaboration and information sharing [16]. Additionally, social media allows for the mass transmission of information at rapid rates. Social network sites are web-based services that allow individuals to create a sharable profile, form a list of other users with whom they share a connection, and share their list of connections and view the lists of others within the system [17]. Through social network sites, once remote communities are connected and able to share information in real time.

Data from the Pew Research Center demonstrated that Facebook is the most popular social networking platform, an estimates 68% of all United States adults and 79% of online adults were using this site in 2016 [18]. While the highest use of

Facebook in online adults is attributed to young adults (88%), there is significant use by many vulnerable demographic groups including low income population (84%), those with lower than a high school education (77%), and Americans living in rural areas (81%) [18]. A popular social network site such as Facebook has the potential to bolster public health education efforts by reaching a high percentage of the United States population. Additionally, social sites are beneficial in providing (1) increased interactions with others, (2) additional available, shared, and tailored information, (3) increased accessibility and widening access to health information, (4) peer/social/emotional support, (5) public health surveillance, and (6) potential to influence health policy [19].

In particular, social networks have been particularly beneficial in chronic conditions such as breast and colorectal cancer and diabetes where active support systems have formed [20]. Studies of the use of social media found that many patients with inflammatory bowel disease (IBD) are interested in receiving disease information from their gastroenterologist and from patient-related organizations via social media [21]. In patients with chronic conditions who are more likely to lack support or access to information, such as those who reside in rural regions, social media provides the potential for cost effective and a wide-reaching form of communication. Another example of high-risk populations who can benefit from social media are adolescents engaged in sexually risky behaviors. Adolescents often lack reliable sources of information due to fear of talking to their parents or lack of resources. Social media can increase knowledge regarding prevention of sexually transmitted diseases (STD), provide physician recommendations on timing of screening and testing and potentially reduce the number of STDs [22]. An additional benefit of social media is the potential to recruit high risk patients for clinical research. A recent cross-sectional study in Atlanta aimed to survey gay men about their experiences with intimate partner violence [23]. Investigators were able to enroll nearly 100 participants through Facebook [23]. While data is often limited in specific populations due to possible stigmas or the inability to reach the population, social campaigns can cross this barrier. Finally, the public health community is increasingly recognizing the potential benefits of social media in disasters. Social media sites are an efficient way to communicate disaster preparedness information with at risk communities as well as a means of responding to those affected during and after the event [24]. In the aftermath of Hurricane Harvey in 2017, Houston and the surrounding areas experienced historic floods. Residents, including those with infants and young children, climbed to their roofs to escape the rising waters, but when some residents were unable to reach emergency services through 911, they requested help on social media sites such as Facebook, Twitter and Nextdoor. Neighbors, rescue volunteers and emergency personnel were able to locate these endangered citizen [25]. While local offices of emergency management are unable to monitor social media sites and discouraged residents from relying on this form of communication [26], it did prove useful during this disaster and there is potential to further develop the use of social media in future disasters.

As future interventions explore options to incorporate social media, it is also important to remain aware of the limitations. A systematic review of the limitations of social media for health communication found a lack of reliable information and concerns about the quality of the messages being conveyed [19]. There was a lack of credible sites and increased potential for breaches in confidentiality [19]. The increased use of social media also raises new ethical considerations such as appropriate personal relationships between patients and providers on sites such as Facebook with potential boundary and privacy issues in the provider-patient context [27]. Healthcare professionals must also be wary of the information they share about their patient interactions. Physician trainees are increasingly exposed to social media training as part of their medical education.

Overall, social media has the potential to provide peer support groups, the sharing of timely information, engage high risk populations on a large scale and has the potential to benefit communities during disaster events. Several limitations to social media exist including lack of quality information and concerns about confidentiality. However, future public health education efforts can continue working to minimize these limitations and maximize the benefits of social sites. Public policies should continue to support increased internet and smart phone access, particularly in low income and rural populations.

The next type of technology that may improve health in disadvantaged populations is telehealth. While telemedicine uses information technology, video imaging and telecommunication to facilitate doctors providing clinical services at a distance, telehealth compasses additional non-physician services [28]. Telehealth has been used to provide services such as subspecialty care, mental health therapies, and most recently, critical care services. Subspecialty telemedicine services have particularly gained success in areas where ability to perform care is less dependent on proximity to the patient. For example, a radiology group with not only a greater quantity of physicians but also more subspecialized services within radiology can review images remotely in a timely manner and provide expertise not otherwise available in rural communities [29]. Telemedicine services also have applications in low-resource patient populations in the treatment of mental health conditions. Among cited barriers to economically disadvantaged populations accessing mental health services are cost, access, and stigma, and, as such, telehealth psychotherapy services for mental health conditions is a particularly promising area for growth. A study of low-income, homebound adults over 50, found that telehealth delivery of problem-solving therapy for depression was as effective as in-person therapy, and the effects of telemedicine were sustained significantly longer [30, 31]. Similarly, economically disadvantaged mothers with young children demonstrated significantly greater reduction in depression after internet-facilitated cognitive-behavioral treatment compared to motivational interviewing and referral to services [32]. Most recently, the growth of intensive and critical care needs has lead to innovation in the use of telehealth. Tele-intensive care unit technologies use teams of intensivist physicians and nurses, who monitor vitals, laboratory results, imaging and medications remotely. This allows them to provide primary physicians on the ground with direct consultations [29]. This decreases overall resource utilization by managing lower severity and lower complexity cases locally and only transferring patients to larger centers if they are critically ill or in need of access to specialized resources.

Overall, telehealth is a growing field and has the potential to improve health outcomes in disadvantaged populations. However, the healthcare system must still proceed with caution. Several potential barriers such as reimbursement negotiations and physician licensing across states are still being addressed. Evidence-based practice will also be essential. In services where telehealth outcomes are not equivalent to in-person options, preference should still be given to the more efficacious treatment options. Otherwise, there is a risk in providing increasingly inequitable care to the most vulnerable populations and widening health disparity gaps. A multi-sector collaboration between the public health community, physicians, managed care organizations, and healthcare policy experts can help ensure the maximization of quality care options reaching these at risk populations.

Mobile computing and communication technologies, social media, and telemedicine are current technology-based strategies which have demonstrated positive outcomes in disparate populations. The future directions of healthcare disparity work must continue to focus on innovative ways to achieve equitable care.

References

1. Falling through the Net: toward digital inclusion: a report on Americans' access to technology tools. US Department of Commerce, Economic and Statistics Administration. 2000.
2. Computer and Internet use in the United States: 2010. http://census.gov/data/tables/2010/demo/computer-internet/computer-use-2010.html. Accessed 5 Nov 2017.
3. Internet/Broadband Fact Sheet. Pew Research Center. http://www.pewinternet.org/fact-sheet/internet-broadband/. Accessed 25 Oct 2017.
4. Lenhart A, Ling R, Campbell S, Purcell K, Sabri E. Teens and mobile phones. Pew Research Center. 2010.
5. Lenhart A. Teens, social media, and technology overview 2015. Pew Research Center. 2015.
6. Badawy SM, Thompson AA, Liem RI. Technology access and smartphone app preferences for medication adherence in adolescents and young adults with sickle cell disease. Pediatr Blood Cancer. 2016;63:848–52.
7. Crosby LE, Ware RE, Goldstein A, et al. Development and evaluation of iManage: a self-management app co-designed by adolescents with sickle cell disease. Pediatr Blood Cancer. 2017;64:139–45.
8. Burke LE, Ma J, Azar KM, et al. Current science on consumer use of mobile health for cardiovascular disease prevention: a scientific statement from the American Heart Association. Circulation. 2015;132:1157–213.
9. Vodopivec-Jamsek V, de Jongh T, Gurol-Urganci I, Atun R, Car J. Mobile phone messaging for preventive health care. Cochrane Database Syst Rev. 2012;12:CD007457.
10. Hardinge M, Rutter H, Velardo C, et al. Using a mobile health application to support self-management in chronic obstructive pulmonary disease: a six-month cohort study. BMC Med Inform Decis Mak. 2015;15:46.
11. Fu H, McMahon SK, Gross CR, Adam TJ, Wyman JF. Usability and clinical efficacy of diabetes mobile applications for adults with type 2 diabetes: a systematic review. Diabetes Res Clin Pract. 2017;131:70–81.

12. Khaylis A, Yiaslas T, Bergstrom J, Gore-Felton C. A review of efficacious technology-based weight-loss interventions: five key components. Telemed J E Health. 2010;16:931–8.
13. Lin CL, Mistry N, Boneh J, Li H, Lazebnik R. Text message reminders increase appointment adherence in a pediatric clinic: a randomized controlled trial. Int J Pediatr. 2016;2016:8487378.
14. Stockwell MS, Kharbanda EO, Martinez RA, et al. Text4Health: impact of text message reminder-recalls for pediatric and adolescent immunizations. Am J Public Health. 2012;102:e15–21.
15. U.S. Food and Drug Administration. FDA approves new continuous glucose monitor for diabetes. https://health.usnews.com/health-care/articles/2017-09-28/fda-approves-new-continuous-glucose-monitor-for-diabetes. News release, Sept. 29th, 2017.
16. Holt D. Branding in the age of social media. Harvard Business Review. https://hbr.org/2016/03/branding-in-the-age-of-social-media. Accessed 18 June 2017.
17. Ellison NB. Social network sites: definition, history, and scholarship. JCMC. 2007;13(1):210–30.
18. Greenwood SPA, Duggan M. Social media update 2016. Pew Research Center. http://www.pewinternet.org/2016/11/11/social-media-update-2016/. Accessed 15 June 2017.
19. Moorhead SA, Hazlett DE, Harrison L, Carroll JK, Irwin A, Hoving C. A new dimension of health care: systematic review of the uses, benefits, and limitations of social media for health communication. J Med Internet Res. 2013;15:e85.
20. Torre-Diez ID-PF, Anton-Rodriguez M. A content analysis of chronic diseases social groups on Facebook and twitter. Telemed E-Health. 2012;18(6):404–8.
21. Reich J, Guo L, Hall J, et al. A survey of social media use and preferences in patients with inflammatory bowel disease. Inflamm Bowel Dis. 2016;22:2678–87.
22. Jones K, Eathington P, Baldwin K, Sipsma H. The impact of health education transmitted via social media or text messaging on adolescent and young adult risky sexual behavior: a systematic review of the literature. Sex Transm Dis. 2014;41:413–9.
23. Strasser SM, Smith M, Pendrick-Denney D, Boos-Beddington S, Chen K, McCarty F. Feasibility study of social media to reduce intimate partner violence among gay men in metro Atlanta, Georgia. West J Emerg Med. 2012;13:298–304.
24. Houston JB, Hawthorne J, Perreault MF, et al. Social media and disasters: a functional framework for social media use in disaster planning, response, and research. Disasters. 2015;39:1–22.
25. Silverman L. Facebook, Twitter replace 911 calls for stranded in Houston. http://www.npr.org/sections/alltechconsidered/2017/08/28/546831780/texas-police-and-residents-turn-to-social-media-to-communicate-amid-harvey. Accessed 12 Sept 2017.
26. Martinez B, Dailey F, Almario CV, et al. Patient understanding of the risks and benefits of biologic therapies in inflammatory bowel disease: insights from a large-scale analysis of social media platforms. Inflamm Bowel Dis. 2017;23:1057–64.
27. Wiener LCC, Grady C, Merchang M. To friend or not to friend: the use of social media in clinical oncology. J Oncol Pract. 2012;8(2):103–6.
28. Weinstein RS, Lopez AM, Joseph BA, et al. Telemedicine, telehealth, and mobile health applications that work: opportunities and barriers. Am J Med. 2014;127:183–7.
29. Kvedar J, Coye MJ, Everett W. Connected health: a review of technologies and strategies to improve patient care with telemedicine and telehealth. Health Aff (Millwood). 2014;33:194–9.
30. Choi NG, Marti CN, Bruce ML, Hegel MT, Wilson NL, Kunik ME. Six-month postintervention depression and disability outcomes of in-home telehealth problem-solving therapy for depressed, low-income homebound older adults. Depress Anxiety. 2014;31:653–61.
31. Choi NG, Hegel MT, Marti N, Marinucci ML, Sirrianni L, Bruce ML. Telehealth problem-solving therapy for depressed low-income homebound older adults. Am J Geriatr Psychiatry. 2014;22:263–71.
32. Sheeber LB, Feil EG, Seeley JR, et al. Mom-net: evaluation of an internet-facilitated cognitive behavioral intervention for low-income depressed mothers. J Consult Clin Psychol. 2017;85:355–66.

Chapter 5
Pediatric Health Disparities and Place-Based Strategies

Jean L. Raphael

Introduction

Healthy development for children consists of interrelated components such as physical development, social competence, emotional maturity, academic learning, general knowledge, and communication [1]. These exposures have implications for both present health and long-term productivity during adulthood [2–5]. A large body of research demonstrates that environmental factors influence health behaviors and health outcomes [6–11]. Inequities in access to healthy environments lead to disparities in health [12–14]. Residents in resource poor neighborhoods typically experience inadequate housing, noise, air pollution, and violent crime which all contribute to poor health.

As researchers and policy makers have increasingly focused on the social determinants of health as a framework for understanding pediatric health disparities, there has been growing interest in approaches and interventions that change the places people work, live, and play [15]. These strategies, collectively termed place-based programs, have the potential to enhance prevention efforts and promote population health. The scientific premise for place-based programs is that public health interventions targeted towards individual behavior, or individuals in general, have limited impact on health. These interventions are often episodic in nature and may disappear when funding is no longer available or sustainable. They may also target a limited number of people or populations. Lastly, they minimize or ignore the social and environmental factors well documented as influencing health [16].

J. L. Raphael (✉)
Pediatrics-Academic General, Baylor College of Medicine, Houston, TX, USA

Influence of Neighborhood on Child Health

A large body of research has explored the influence of neighborhood environment on child health and development [17]. Many have collectively focused on factors related to disadvantage (e.g., income, employment, occupation status, family structure, racial/ethnic diversity, residential stability). These studies have demonstrated that disadvantage tends to be geographically concentrated. With respect to child health, neighborhood disadvantage has been adversely associated with children's learning, academic performance, and social, emotional, and behavioral outcomes. In addition to markers of disadvantage, other factors have been explored for their impact on children's developmental outcomes. Neighborhood stressors (e.g., crime) and social organization (social capital, collective efficacy) also influence children's developmental outcomes. Increased neighborhood social capital and collective efficacy have been associated with positive child development and behavioral outcomes. There is also data that supports the importance of the built environment in child health outcomes [7, 8]. Physical features such as housing density, neighborhood destinations, green space, and traffic exposure have all been studied as influences.

Increasingly, researchers are improving the science in linking neighborhood environment measures with existing child health outcomes. Neighborhood factors can be measured subjectively (e.g., surveys) or objectively (spatial measures). The availability of spatial software such as Geographic Information Systems (GIS) has facilitated more advanced analyses [17]. Spatial datasets may measure destinations and services, street network, and park attributes [18]. They can be linked to child outcomes with accurate information on where the child lives. Typical spatial boundaries used to define neighborhoods include cities, suburbs, census tracts, and school areas. However, these boundaries may not reflect the true neighborhood the child and family experience [17]. Therefore, it is also important to collect information on parental and child perceptions of neighborhood (e.g., perceived crime, perceived access to destinations). Integrating subjective and objective measures may offer new capabilities to determine whether interventions should target the environment, perceptions, or both simultaneously.

Definition of Place-Based Approaches

Place is characterized by infrastructure such as school, hospitals, recreational facilities, retail outlets, and housing [19]. Healthier environments are made possible by health-promoting amenities such as maintained homes, parks, safe walking paths, and full-service grocery stores. Place-based approaches (PBAs) are gaining widespread support among policy makers as a mechanism to improve population health and reduce health disparities. PBAs are defined as a collaborative strategy to address complex social-economic issues through interventions localized to a specific geographic scale [19–21]. Specific terms for these approaches include comprehensive community initiatives, collaborative environmental management, community economic development, collective impact initiates, and complex adaptive systems [16]. Despite the differences in nomenclature, they share high-level commonalities in both purpose and implementation. PBAs target an entire community rather than focusing principally on problems faced by individuals [22]. Their overall objectives consist of empowering the community, improving service delivery and coordination, improving particular social objectives, and improving whole communities. They specifically aim to address issues such as poor housing, social isolation, fragmented service delivery, and limited economic opportunities. Overall PBAs should have three major features—structural changes to places, scalability, and sustainability over time. Programs and interventions that focus on structural factors have the potential to impact larger populations for longer periods of time than those focusing on individuals. Basic structures producing negative health in people's surroundings must be changed in order to facilitate transformational improvements. Scalability is also important in terms of maximizing the reach of a particular program. Initiatives should not be overly complex or costly if they are to be scaled up and reproduced in other regions or communities. Sustainability is important in ensuring that programs continue to exist after initial input of intellectual and financial resources. Other key characteristics of PBAs include targeting a specific geographic area, engaging multi-sector stakeholders, leveraging local knowledge and assets, enabling stakeholder ownership of the initiative, and promoting flexibility and adaptability in design. Stakeholders involved in PBAs may include government officials, business, non-profit organizations, and individual citizens. It is postulated that PBAs can foster change in a number of areas. Such initiatives have the potential to improve economic opportunity, enhance the quality of schools, lead to more open green space, promote healthier food options, and improved access to care.

Rationale for PBAs to Address Child Health Disparities

The emergence of PBAs as a strategy to address disparities in child health stems from a number of factors [22]. A large body of research demonstrates that physical and social environments influence health and wellbeing [17]. The daily experiences of children within these environments determine health outcomes over time. Social networks also impact wellbeing. Children exist within families and a broader community where social support or isolation can influence child development. Disadvantage at the level of local communities (e.g., low school attainment, high unemployment rate, poor health, high imprison rate, child abuse, domestic violence) can lead to intergenerational disadvantage.

In addition to these environmental challenges, traditional approaches to reduce inequities have failed to produce substantial improvements in the health of children. Such strategies have included making existing health care services more accessible and implementing behavior change interventions at the level of individuals. However they do not typically address root causes of inequities, predominantly focus on treatment rather than prevention, require significant time investment for target populations, and fail to produce long-term and sustainable change [16, 22]. Many local services and community-based agencies are unable to adequately support families because needs are often complex and change over time. With developmental changes, a child's needs will evolve over time. Lastly, it is frequently difficult to engage and retain vulnerable families in services or interventions. Even when in need, families may not use available services. Reasons for poor engagement include lack of awareness regarding services, difficulty navigating a fragmented service system, inability to access services, or competing priorities. Taken together, these factors provide a strong rationale for PBAs.

Challenges to Assessing Place-Based Approaches

Researchers have had difficulty in assessing the efficacy and effectiveness of PBAs as outcome evaluations for them are lacking [16, 19]. Many of the key characteristics shared by different PBA models are difficult to operationalize or measure in evaluations. Much of these challenges occur because PBAs occur in open systems [16]. PBA efforts are multi-faceted, working across diverse sectors, such as health, education, and housing. Consequently, disentangling the effects of individual strategies is challenging in evaluation. Another challenge of PBAs relates to dosage. These types of interventions are flexible and assumed to evolve over time in response to changes in the locally targeted community. Therefore, tracking consistency of dosage over time is difficult. At the same time, the reach and dosage of some interventions may not be evenly distributed throughout the target community. Differences in dosage may vary across residents, neighborhoods, or organizations.

These challenges raise numerous tensions among stakeholders invested in the implementation of PBAs [16, 23]. The first tension consists within the evaluation field about how to measure impact. There have been debates about the best research designs for PBAs that have the ability to estimate causal effects. While some researchers advocate randomized control trials (RCTs) with random assignment of treatment and control interventions, opponents argue that these designs are not the sole strategy for determining impact and that such approaches may not be ethical in working with vulnerable communities. The second tension that may occur exists between evaluators and practitioners. Community development practitioners are invested in implementing change as soon as possible. Quick successes, small or early, enhance cross-sector collaborations and leverages existing resources that may be uncertain in the future. Unfortunately, changes in community conditions, as outcomes of PBAs, may not take place for years. Some changes are difficult to assess or detect. While practitioners may see impact according to their experience of the community, evaluators may not be able to provide corresponding data to demonstrate effectiveness. As an example, community capacity is typically a priority outcome in PBAs. However, no definitive measures of capacity exist. Consequently, evaluation options are intensive with respect to both time and resources. This conflict between research and action may compromise efforts to successfully implement PBAs.

A third tension may exist between evaluators and funders regarding objectivity. Evaluators for PBAs are tasked with carrying out independent, neutral research but may be drawn into various roles with the interventions, compromising their role as an external researcher. As standard for program evaluation, evaluators are incorporated into the early stages of program development. This early involvement allows the evaluators to gain an accurate assessment of the baseline for observing subsequent changes. Evaluators may then be involved with numerous steps in the intervention, including technical assistance with ongoing data collection and formative and summative evaluation activities determining how a program unfolds in real time. The multiple roles of evaluators may bring them in close proximity to the process of planning and implementation. This may consist of interactions with community-based organizations, coalition partners, and community members. Given the scope of these interactions, it is possible that evaluators may become part of the interventions themselves. Funders may find concern in the ability of evaluators to remain neutral and objective over time. Another challenge in evaluation of PBAs lies in the ability to assess long-term objectives. Meaningful outcomes for complex problems may not be realized for decades and therefore often lie outside the time frame of programs and their evaluation assessments. Evaluations are typically limited to their specific funding periods. Short time frames can lead to narrow evaluations that miss critical benefits, underestimate costs, or fail to capture sustainability. Lastly, evaluation of PBAs may be complicated by availability of data. In many cases, PBAs may receive financial support from multiple funders. Funders may have different objectives and desired outcomes, thus creating a burden on measurement. This leads to conflict on what outcomes to measure and how they should be measured. Data collected by one partner may not align with the needs of other partners in the initiative.

Effectiveness of Place-Based Approaches

Establishing an evidence base for PBAs requires developing an understanding of what proves success [16, 19, 22]. Positive findings associated with PBAs focused on child health have been at the levels of *individuals in the target community* (e.g., increased access to services, reduction in inequities), *professionals* (e.g., enhanced knowledge, improved skills, better understanding of children's needs, job satisfaction, leadership), *agencies* (e.g., improved efficiency), and *communities* (e.g., enhanced capacity building). Negative outcomes associated with PBAs have included increased workload for professionals and agencies in the short-term and increased demand for services as a result of needs being identified earlier. A number of reviews have provided evidence on the enablers of effective PBAs (Table 5.1) [16, 19, 22].

Table 5.1 Characteristics of successful place-based approaches

Characteristic	Description
Age span	• Initiative targets a specific and well-defined age or developmental period
Defined geographic area	• Program focuses on a specific community or region
Multi-level approach	• Program intervenes at three or more levels of influence
Active community participation, engagement, and leadership	• Communities provide maximum input • Communities have decisional authority
Investment in capacity building	• Adequate time and resources provided for communities • Intervention staff integrated into long-term efforts
Sufficient time	• Adequate time built into program for behavior change
Adequate funding	• Government provides core public infrastructure • Private sector funds leveraged to support initiatives
Strong government leadership and support	• Government consistently articulates support • Government acts as partner in efforts
Effective relationships between stakeholders	• High levels of trust and communication • Shared vision and values
Good fit	• Scale of project appropriate for policy challenge • Community prepared to implement the intervention • Intervention meets the needs of the community • Intervention appropriate for targeted cultural groups
Backbone organization	• Separate organization has its own staff and specific set of skills to serve as backbone for the entire initiative • This organization coordinates participating agencies

Evolution of Place-Based Approaches

Models of PBAs have evolved in the United States. Collective impact initiatives gained prominence over the past several years [16, 19, 22]. These models are based on shared efforts between philanthropy, community services, and businesses. Typically, collective impact initiatives employ a "cradle to career" approach focused on addressing all the factors that impact child health from birth to adulthood.

Several collective impact initiatives specific to children have come to prominence (Table 5.2) [19].

PBAs vs. Person-Based Approaches

While PBAs offer numerous benefits, they only represent one policy-oriented strategy to reduce health disparities among children [16, 19, 22]. PBAs represent an option that policy-makers and public managers may select based on existing evidence about knowledge of current conditions and expected outcomes. In some cases, a person-based approach may be more appropriate. Such approaches may be preferred when addressing a health issue with a relatively straight-forward known cause and evidence-based interventions. PBAs are more appropriate for complex

Table 5.2 Model community impact initiatives specific to children

Program	Characteristics
Harlem children's zone	• Established in 1990s • Goal to improve lives of poor children in New York • 97 block community service project • Includes charter schools, social services, parenting classes, early childhood development program, after school program
Strive partnership of Cincinnati	• Established in 2006 • Goal to improve outcomes for children and families • Cradle-to-Career program committed to improving child educational outcomes • Voluntary partnership of hundreds of organizations
Magnolia place community initiative	• Established in 2008 • Goal to improve health, educational, social, and economic outcomes of children living in the 500-block Magnolia catchment area in Los Angeles • Involves over 70 community organizations, schools, businesses, and local government agencies
Promise neighborhoods	• Established in 2010 by US Department of Education • Competitive program awards • Goal to improve outcomes for children through cradle-to-career services • Targets children and families in underserved areas

problems for which the solutions are uncertain or require multiple forms of intervention.

In this chapter, we have summarized the potential of PBAs to address disparities in pediatric health. While the potential is great, the challenges to implementation and evaluation are complex and occur at a number of levels. The existing evidence base on PBAs speak to the promise and peril of these interventions. Future priorities for this field will consist of further establishment of the evidence base, development of evaluation tools, and cost-effectiveness assessment.

References

1. Shonkoff JP, Richter L, van der Gaag J, Bhutta ZA. An integrated scientific framework for child survival and early childhood development. Pediatrics. 2012;129:e460–72.
2. Case A, Fertig A, Paxson C. The lasting impact of childhood health and circumstance. J Health Econ. 2005;24:365–89.
3. Heckman JJ. Skill formation and the economics of investing in disadvantaged children. Science. 2006;312:1900–2.
4. Lu MC, Halfon N. Racial and ethnic disparities in birth outcomes: a life-course perspective. Matern Child Health J. 2003;7:13–30.
5. Braveman P, Barclay C. Health disparities beginning in childhood: a life-course perspective. Pediatrics. 2009;124(Suppl 3):S163–75.
6. Morenoff JD. Neighborhood mechanisms and the spatial dynamics of birth weight. AJS Am J Sociol. 2003;108:976–1017.

7. Sallis JF, Floyd MF, Rodriguez DA, Saelens BE. Role of built environments in physical activity, obesity, and cardiovascular disease. Circulation. 2012;125:729–37.
8. Ding D, Gebel K. Built environment, physical activity, and obesity: what have we learned from reviewing the literature? Health Place. 2012;18:100–5.
9. Galvez MP, McGovern K, Knuff C, et al. Associations between neighborhood resources and physical activity in inner-city minority children. Acad Pediatr. 2013;13:20–6.
10. Carlson JA, Saelens BE, Kerr J, et al. Association between neighborhood walkability and GPS-measured walking, bicycling and vehicle time in adolescents. Health Place. 2015;32:1–7.
11. Diez Roux AV. Integrating social and biologic factors in health research: a systems view. Ann Epidemiol. 2007;17:569–74.
12. Lantz PM, House JS, Lepkowski JM, Williams DR, Mero RP, Chen J. Socioeconomic factors, health behaviors, and mortality: results from a nationally representative prospective study of US adults. JAMA. 1998;279:1703–8.
13. Sorlie PD, Backlund E, Keller JB. US mortality by economic, demographic, and social characteristics: the National Longitudinal Mortality Study. Am J Public Health. 1995;85:949–56.
14. Andrulis DP. Access to care is the centerpiece in the elimination of socioeconomic disparities in health. Ann Intern Med. 1998;129:412–6.
15. CSDH. Closing the gap in a generation: health equity through action on the social determinants of health. Final report of the Commission on Social Determinants of Health. Geneva: World Health Organization; 2008.
16. Bellefontaine T, Wisener R. The evaluation of place-based approaches: questions for further research. Ottawa: Policy Horizons Canada; 2011.
17. Villanueva K, Badland H, Kvalsvig A, et al. Can the neighborhood built environment make a difference in children's development? Building the research agenda to create evidence for place-based children's policy. Acad Pediatr. 2016;16:10–9.
18. Villanueva K, Badland H, Giles-Corti B, Goldfeld S. Using spatial analysis of the Australian Early Development Index to advance our understanding of 'neighbourhood effects' research on child health and development. J Paediatr Child Health. 2015;51:577–9.
19. Moore TG, McHugh-Dilloon H, Bull K, Fry R, Laidlow B, West S. The evidence: what we know about place-based approaches to support children's well-being. Parkville: Murdoch Children's Research Institute and The Royal Children's Hospital Centre for Community Child Health; 2014.
20. Dupre ME, Moody J, Nelson A, et al. Place-based initiatives to improve health in disadvantaged communities: cross-sector characteristics and networks of local actors in North Carolina. Am J Public Health. 2016;106:1548–55.
21. Vechakul J, Shrimali BP, Sandhu JS. Human-centered design as an approach for place-based innovation in public health: a case study from Oakland, California. Matern Child Health J. 2015;19:2552–9.
22. Place-based approaches to supporting children and families. The Royal Children's Hospital Centre for Community Child Health. 2011.
23. Dillman K, Peck LR. Tensions and opportunities in evaluating place-based interventions. Community Invest. 2012;24:15–7.

Chapter 6
Healthcare Financing and Social Determinants

Jean L. Raphael

Introduction

As health care continues to advance along the principles of the Triple Aim with a reimbursement model of value-based care [1], there has been increasing call to include social determinants of health (SDH) in reform strategies [2]. An extensive body of evidence demonstrates that SDH play a substantial role in shaping health and health outcomes and addressing disparities [3–12]. Growing recognition of the benefits of connecting health care with non-health services has led to major initiatives focused on addressing SDH [13, 14]. Some states have implemented a "Health in All Policies Approach", which prioritizes health as a key outcome of policymaking across sectors [15]. Private organizations and foundations have begun to address SDH through community partnerships and funding priorities [16]. However, the health care system does not routinely or systematically collect SDH data or coordinate care to address social needs. It also does not regularly reimburse providers for addressing SDH. The emerging question is how health care financing can be aligned to promote health equity through addressing SDH. The goal of this chapter is to describe the role of health care financing in addressing SDH, and in turn, health disparities among children.

J. L. Raphael (✉)
Pediatrics-Academic General, Baylor College of Medicine, Houston, TX, USA

The Potential of Medicaid to Address SDH

For children specifically, the role of Medicaid in addressing SDH is particularly important. Medicaid and the Children's Health Insurance Program (CHIP) cover nearly 45% of children under the age of 6, and nearly half of all births in the United States [17]. Therefore, Medicaid has major capacity to influence how SDH can be incorporated into health care financing for children. Medicaid programs are uniquely positioned to bridge the gap between health care and non-health services that have the potential to improve health outcomes [18]. First, Medicaid has the infrastructure to develop a model of integrated health and social service system. With a model of state-federal partnership, Medicaid programs can be customized to meet the unique need of each state's populations and circumstances, and can foster collaborations between state and federal agencies. Medicaid serves over 74 million beneficiaries and therefore can assess eligibility and needs based on a variety of demographic factors [18]. Medicaid serves many of the individuals, specifically children, who can benefit the most from non- health services and interventions that address SDH. Lastly, there is a strong business case for Medicaid to address SDH. Strategies to address SDH in combination with timely access to care, behavioral health, and home and community-based services can reduce unnecessary and potentially expensive medical care. States can use Medicaid to remove barriers between the health care system and other sectors to promote health and well-being. New payment models that make providers accountable for patient health and costs of treatment through shared savings, global budgets, and capitated payments also provide impetus for clinicians to address non health care factors.

The move specifically towards value-based payment has created policy opportunities to address SDH [2, 19]. The general rationale to account for SDH in quality improvement and payment policies is that such action would provide Medicaid with improved understanding of quality across providers and populations and more accurate payments. Data on how SDH influence cost and quality of care could help Medicaid develop strategies to better address disparities in a cost-effective manner. State Medicaid programs have multiple reasons to incorporate SDH data into their quality improvement initiatives. States that adjust for SDH in making quality comparisons across plans have the potential to develop more accurate and meaningful comparisons among plans [2]. A deeper understanding of variations in quality across Medicaid populations and subpopulations can inform new programs to address gaps in quality. Separately accounting for SDH in Medicaid payment models may create better alignment between the risk of the population and the payment amount. The overall goal would be payment that realistically reflects the health and well-being of the population and their likely health care and social service needs [2]. A more accurate payment model would help Medicaid health plans design the right incentives and help them formulate strategies to meet the needs of covered populations. More globally, such an approach would ensure that taxpayer money is used more effectively.

States have not historically accounted for SDH in Medicaid payment models. More typically, states set capitation rates and total costs of care targets for Medicaid plans using only diagnosis-based risk adjustment to determine the relative risk of a plan's Medicaid population. These relative risk scores do not account for SDH such as income, education, or housing status [2]. Without adjustment for SDH in payment models, states may financially penalize managed care organizations for caring for children with substantial social challenges or designing unique programs to address the needs of these individuals. By adjusting payments for SDH, states can effectively support health plans and providers to innovate and create novel, tailored services for children who experience poor outcomes.

Medicaid Policies That Promote Addressing SDH

Historically, several Medicaid programs have facilitated opportunities to address SDH [18]. The Delivery System Reform Incentive Program (DSRIP) mandates states to reduce hospitalizations, improve outcomes, and convert Medicaid providers to value-based contracts. Under Section 1115 of the Social Security Act, Medicaid programs can transform state health care systems through DSRIP. Such transformation may include "infrastructure development, system redesign, clinical outcome improvement, and population-focused improvements." Several states have used the 1115 waiver to address SDH. Oregon used Medicaid funding for health-related supportive services such as education, job training, and support groups. New York has addressed SDH through its Medicaid Redesign Team (MRT). It has used its Medicaid dollars to fund job training, rental subsidy assistance, and tenant support to reduce preventable hospitalizations.

Revised managed care regulations have enhanced Medicaid's ability to invest in initiatives that address SDH and improve population health [20]. Most recently in 2016, the Centers for Medicare and Medicaid Services (CMS) updated Medicaid managed care regulations. Since the last update in 2002, managed care has become the predominant Medicaid delivery model [20]. In updating the managed care regulations, CMS sought to promote practices and models of care that went beyond clinical care to address social and structural factors that impact health and health outcomes. Several new regulations have the potential to support addressing SDH.

Alternative Payment Models to Pay Providers

The regulations formalize mechanisms for states to implement incentive-based payment systems for managed care organizations. They allow states to require managed care entities to implement alternative payment models (APMs) for their providers [20]. APMs have emerged as a mechanism to account for SDH and support providers in advancing quality, patient outcomes, and cost reduction. The new regulations reduce administrative obstacles and thereby promote future implementation. States now have the ability to leverage APMs to invest in community-level health interventions. States may encourage or require specific APMs, including models that connect health with non-health services. This may include screenings for SDH such as food insecurity, domestic abuse, and environmental hazards in the home. The goal of such screenings would be to identify and address factors that increase health risks or compromise medical management.

Medicaid should follow specific principles in order to design and assess APMs that revolve around SDH. The American Academy of Family Physicians has outlined five principles to address SDH in APMs: (1) APMs should support practices' efforts to identify and address SDH that are shown to impact health outcomes; (2) The incorporation of variables representing SDH should be founded on evidence-based research methods; (3) Health information technology (HIT) platforms should facilitate SDH data collection from medical records and other sources to support improved clinical decision making, care coordination, quality measurement, and population health management; (4) To minimize administrative burden on providers and patients, SDH data should be collected by leveraging existing mechanisms; and (5) To ensure APMs improve access, quality, and health equity, practices should receive appropriate resources and support to identify, monitor, and assess SDH [19].

Incentivize Health Plans to Invest

Under a separate provision of the revised CMS managed care regulations, states were given the ability to design payment incentives for health plans, including establishment of performance benchmarks related to addressing SDH [20]. For example, a state could withhold part of a health plan's capitation rate unless it surpasses a state-set goal for improving lead screening for young children.

Nontraditional Services

Historically Medicaid managed care plans have had the capacity to pay for nontraditional services outside contractual obligations. This policy allows plans the flexibility to apply simple solutions towards the problems of beneficiaries [20]. These extra services are categorized as "in-lieu-of" services and "value-added" services. An "in-lieu-of" service is one that substitutes for a similar service covered under the contract. For example, a typical prenatal visit could be substituted for a home visit for pregnant mothers to provide preventive care. The new regulations clarify that such in-lieu-of service expenditures qualify as covered services for rate setting. Value-added services are extra services unrelated to contracted services. Examples include nutrition classes and peer-support services. These services give health plans flexibility to address social needs beyond what is defined in the Medicaid state plan.

Challenges to Incorporating SDH into Medicaid Policies

While increasing awareness and changes in Medicaid regulations have advanced models of using health care financing to address SDH, conceptual and logistical challenges remain [20].

Adjusting performance measurement by SDH has some potential drawbacks. If not designed properly, adjustment models could in some cases create unwanted incentives by inappropriately increasing the performance scores of providers treating vulnerable children. Downward adjustments in performance benchmarks would acknowledge the role of SDH play in shaping health outcomes. Downward adjustment would also protect health plans from being penalized for failing to hit performance targets. Conversely, a state that adjusts quality performance expectations for SDH may inadvertently create a tiered system that perpetuates disparities by having different benchmarks for different providers. Plans and providers may be enabled to provide poorer care (e.g., fewer immunizations, less developmental screenings) to beneficiaries with more adverse social circumstances.

Innovative programs advanced through Medicaid to address SDH may bring Return on Investment (ROI) but not necessarily in the health care sector. For example, a program that increases access to behavioral health may save money and reduce incarceration. In this case, the managed care organization invests substantially, the criminal justice contributes less, and the ultimate benefit goes to society. Health plans must find ways to create effective and sustainable population health initiatives that distribute savings across sectors such that the health plan also experiences benefit.

In child health, the benefits of specific investments may not be realized for years. The ROI from a program addressing SDH impacting obesity may not manifest for years. Sustained coverage and long horizons for ROI are critical to creating a model where both the enrollee and health plan benefit from the initial investment.

Another potential challenge is that programs become so successful they adversely impact the finances of the health plan in the future [18]. In this way, programs become victims of their own success. As an example, a managed care organization may initiate a program to implement environmental controls in the homes of children with asthma. This program may decrease asthma-related emergency department encounters and hospitalizations and thereby produce immediate savings. However, the reduced spending might lower the plan's capitation rates in subsequent years. Long term, health plans may be disincentivized to engage in value-based payment initiatives.

As Medicaid has grown and evolved to meet the Triple Aim of Health Care, it has advanced its model of care and reimbursement beyond traditional health care only paradigms of care. New innovations in Medicaid supported by changes in Medicaid policy have enabled states to invest in novel programs to address SDH and improve population health. Ultimately, Medicaid cannot reform care models on its own. Commercial payers must also contribute to bridging the connections between health and non-health services. However, Medicaid can continue to model innovation and best practices and thereby foster more effective health care delivery.

References

1. Berwick DM, Nolan TW, Whittington J. The triple aim: care, health, and cost. Health Aff. 2008;27:759–69.
2. Breslin E, Lambertino A, Heaphy D. Medicaid and social determinants of health: adjusting payment and measuring health outcomes. At https://www.healthmanagement.com/wp-content/uploads/SHVS_SocialDeterminants_HMA_July2017.pdf.
3. Beal AC. High-quality health care: the essential route to eliminating disparities and achieving health equity. Health Aff. 2011;30:1868–71.
4. Beck AF, Huang B, Ryan PH, Sandel MT, Chen C, Kahn RS. Areas with high rates of police-reported violent crime have higher rates of childhood asthma morbidity. J Pediatr. 2016;173:175–82.e1.
5. Beck AF, Klein MD, Schaffzin JK, Tallent V, Gillam M, Kahn RS. Identifying and treating a substandard housing cluster using a medical-legal partnership. Pediatrics. 2012;130:831–8.
6. Beck AF, Simmons JM, Huang B, Kahn RS. Geomedicine: area-based socioeconomic measures for assessing risk of hospital reutilization among children admitted for asthma. Am J Public Health. 2012;102:2308–14.
7. Bloomberg GR, Trinkaus KM, Fisher EB Jr, Musick JR, Strunk RC. Hospital readmissions for childhood asthma: a 10-year metropolitan study. Am J Respir Crit Care Med. 2003;167:1068–76.
8. Braveman P, Barclay C. Health disparities beginning in childhood: a life-course perspective. Pediatrics. 2009;124(Suppl 3):S163–75.
9. Carlson JA, Saelens BE, Kerr J, et al. Association between neighborhood walkability and GPS-measured walking, bicycling and vehicle time in adolescents. Health Place. 2015;32:1–7.
10. Case A, Fertig A, Paxson C. The lasting impact of childhood health and circumstance. J Health Econ. 2005;24:365–89.
11. Flores G, Committee On Pediatric R. Technical report – racial and ethnic disparities in the health and health care of children. Pediatrics. 2010;125:e979–e1020.
12. Hasnain-Wynia R, Baker DW, Nerenz D, et al. Disparities in health care are driven by where minority patients seek care: examination of the hospital quality alliance measures. Arch Intern Med. 2007;167:1233–9.
13. Dupre ME, Moody J, Nelson A, et al. Place-based initiatives to improve health in disadvantaged communities: cross-sector characteristics and networks of local actors in North Carolina. Am J Public Health. 2016;106:1548–55.
14. Place-based approaches to supporting children and families. The Royal Children's Hospital Centre for Community Child Health. 2011.
15. Rigby E, Hatch ME. Incorporating economic policy into a 'health-in-all-policies' agenda. Health Aff. 2016;35:2044–52.
16. Isham GJ, Zimmerman DJ, Kindig DA, Hornseth GW. HealthPartners adopts community business model to deepen focus on nonclinical factors of health outcomes. Health Aff. 2013;32:1446–52.
17. Smith VK, Gifford K, Ellis E, Edwards B. Implementing coverage and payment initiatives: results from a 50-state Medicaid budget survey for state fiscal years 2016 and 2017. The Henry J. Kaiser Family Foundation. At http://files.kff.org/attachment/Report-Implementing-Coverage-and-Payment-Initiatives. Accessed 4 Sept 2018.
18. National Quality Forum. A framework for Medicaid programs to address social determinants of health: food insecurity and housing instability. http://www.qualityforum.org/Publications/2017/12/Food_Insecurity_and_Housing_Instability_Final_Report.aspx
19. Advancing health equity: principles to address the social determinants of health in alternative payment models. https://www.aafp.org/about/policies/all/socialdeterminants-paymentmodels.html
20. Machledt D. Addressing the social determinants of health through Medicaid managed care. https://www.commonwealthfund.org/publications/issue-briefs/2017/nov/addressing-social-determinants-healththrough-medicaid-managed

Chapter 7
Future Directions for a Solutions-Based Approach

Jean L. Raphael

Introduction

As disparities in child health continue to be persistent and pervasive, clinicians, health care delivery systems, and policymakers share a collective responsibility to develop, implement, and evaluate innovative solutions. Inequities in child health represent both an economic and ethical imperative. Since the publication of *Unequal Treatment*, a large body of research documenting inequities has developed in the adult literature with subsequent emergence of such work in pediatrics. Over time, researchers and policymakers have increasingly demonstrated the impact of disparities over the life-course [1]. Disparities that originate in childhood are associated with adult chronic disease. More broadly, one's experiences in childhood can influence patterns of disease, aging, and mortality later in life [2]. Life-course science is placing an increasing responsibility on pediatric practice and research to more effectively prevent and manage the childhood precursors of adult-onset disease. Given these linkages, there is urgent need to study health inequities in child health and how solutions enacted during childhood may impact adult health, well-being, and long-term productivity. Future advancements must be developed and cultivated along the pillars of clinical care, research, and policy.

J. L. Raphael (✉)
Pediatrics-Academic General, Baylor College of Medicine, Houston, TX, USA

While large-scale solutions at the level of population health are clearly warranted to address inequities in child health, the intimate and long-term clinician-patient relationship provides a unique opportunity to discover and address the root causes of disparities. Health system investment is required to support practice innovation towards achieving health equity. A paper by Cheng et al. provides a comprehensive roadmap of how pediatric clinicians supported by health systems can assess and address health disparities in practice [3]. Strategies described include culturally competent care, systematic and routine review of both practice performance data and population health data, periodic conduct of community needs assessments, development of family advisory boards to ensure feedback on care systems, screening for social determinants of health with provision of community resources, recognition of health literacy challenges, acknowledgement of implicit bias in care, commitment to workforce diversity, and involvement in advocacy.

Research efforts to address disparities must increasingly target development of interventions specific to children. While the root causes of health disparities are complex and continue to warrant investigation, investments must also be focused towards solutions-based strategies across the continuum of research investigation (basic science, translational, clinical, health services, comparative effectiveness research) and quality improvement. Innovative methodological approaches must be promoted to overcome the historical limitations of health disparities research. This will require both investment and calculated risk on the parts of large funding agencies such as the National Institutes of Health, Agency for Healthcare Research and Quality, Patient Centered Outcomes Research Institute, and Robert Wood Johnson Foundation. Wherever possible, research should explore the promise of life-course science and opportunities to partner with communities.

Health policy initiatives represent a third key pillar in addressing inequities in child health. Payers, including commercial insurance companies and government, must leverage their roles as decision makers in incentivizing clinicians to focus on child health disparities. Alternative payment models that reimburse pediatricians for screening and addressing social determinants of health have the potential to transform practice. Payment models which risk adjust for social determinants of health may preserve the pediatric workforce in underserved communities. State and federal service grants to address disparities in child health can also play an important role. The federal government has the authority to enforce policies that promote accurate, complete collection of race and ethnicity data to monitor disparities. The government can also set measurable goals for improving quality of care and achieving equity for all underserved subgroups of children with the realization that inequities go beyond historical paradigms limited to race and ethnicity.

References

1. Braveman P, Barclay C. Health disparities beginning in childhood: a life-course perspective. Pediatrics. 2009;124(Suppl 3):S163–75.
2. Wise PH. Child poverty and the promise of human capacity: childhood as a foundation for healthy aging. Acad Pediatr. 2016;16:S37–45.
3. Cheng TL, Emmanuel MA, Levy DJ, Jenkins RR. Child health disparities: what can a clinician do? Pediatrics. 2015;136:961–8.

Index

A

Advocacy, 54
Affordable Care Act, 13, 25, 26
Agency for Healthcare Research and Quality
    (AHRQ), 1, 13
Alternative payment models (APMs), 49
American Academy of Family Physicians, 50
American Indian/Alaska Native (AIAN), 8
American Public Health Association, 25
Asthma, 6–8, 19, 27

B

Backbone organization, 44
Built environment, 3, 40
Business Process Reengineering (BPR), 11

C

Centers for Medicare and Medicaid Services
    (CMS), 26, 49
Children in immigrant families (CIF), 3
Children's Health Insurance Program (CHIP),
    7, 48
Chronic Obstructive Pulmonary Disease, 32
Community, 35, 42, 43
Community environmental specialists
    (CESs), 27
Community health workers (CHWs), 20
    cardiovascular disease, 27
    chronic conditions, 26
    community health, 26
    community organizations, 26
    core competencies, 26
    cost-effective interventions, 27
    evidence-based recommendations, 28
    evidence supports, 26
    health disparities, 25
    Medicaid transport services, 26
    national organizations, 28
    navigator, 25
    peer educator, 25
    public health, 25
    social determinants, 26
    state regulations, 28
    Type II Diabetes, 27
Community needs assessment, 54
Comparative effectiveness research, 54
Continuous glucose monitoring (CGM)
    systems, 33
Continuous Quality Improvement (CQI), 11
Crossing the Quality Chasm, 12
Cultural competency, 5
Culturally competent care, 54

D

Delivery System Reform Incentive Program
    (DSRIP), 49
Demographics of children, 6
Department of State Health Services, 25
Diabetes, 19, 34
Disparity
    adult
        demographics, 6
        dependency, 5, 6
        development, 4
        differential epidemiology, 6
        5 D's and relevance, 4, 5
        health care financing (Dollars), 7

Disparity (*cont.*)
   child health
      access to care, 8
      health service use, 8
      medical status, 8
   definitions, 2
   goals, 2

E
Early intervention, 4
Ethnicity, 3, 7, 8

F
Family advisory boards, 54
Focus, Analyze, Develop, Execute/Evaluate
   (FADE), 11

G
Geographic Information Systems (GIS), 40

H
Health care financing, *see* Social determinants
   of health (SDH)
Health care utilization, 19
Health equity, 4
Health in All Policies Approach, 47
Health information technology (HIT), 50
Health literacy, 15, 54
Health Resources and Services
   Administration, 25
Healthy People 2020, 32

I
Implicit bias, 54
Inflammatory bowel disease (IBD), 34
Infrastructure, 40
Institute of Medicine (IOM), 1, 7, 12
Intergenerational disadvantage, 41
Internet, 31, 32, 35

L
Life-course science, 5, 53, 54
Limited English Proficiency (LEP), 8

M
Measurement fixation, 16
Medicaid, 7
Medicaid Redesign Team (MRT), 49

N
National Center on Minority Health and
   Health Disparities, 1
National Healthcare Quality Report and
   National Healthcare Disparities
   Report, 7
Nextdoor, 34
Nutrition, 16, 50

O
Office of Management and Budget (OMB), 3

P
Patient Centered Outcomes Research Institute
   (PCORI), 20
Patient Protection, 25, 26
Pew Research Center, 31, 33
Place-based approaches (PBAs)
   challenges, 42
   child health, 40, 41
   definition, 40
   effectiveness, 43
   evolution of, 44
   healthy development for children, 39
   influence of neighborhood, 40
   interventions, 39
   vs. person-based approaches, 44
   researchers and policy makers, 39
Plan, Do, Study, Act (PDSA), 11
Poverty, 3, 6
Promotores, 25
Provider profiling, 14
Public health interventions, 39
Public reporting, 14, 16

Q
Quality improvement (QI)
   challenges, 15
   child health, 12
   collaborative, 20, 21
   consideration of comparators, 17
   efficiency, 17, 20
   evidence base, disparities, 14
   health and health care, 11
   implementation, 14, 18, 20
   innovate approaches, 11
   investigators, 18
   leveraging community resources, 20
   mechanism of intervention, 18
   methodological rigor, 18
   performance, 12, 13, 16
   social determinants of health (SDH), 19

R
Race, 3, 7, 8
Randomized control trials (RCTs), 42
Reimbursement model, 47, 51
Return on Investment (ROI), 51
Risk adjustment, 49

S
Scalability, 41
Self management, 32
Sexually transmitted diseases (STD), 34
Sexual orientation, 3, 4, 15, 17
Shared decision making, 8
Sickle cell disease, 33
Social capital, 40
Social determinants of health (SDH), 3, 6
    Medicaid
        APMs, 49
        challenges, 51
        health care and non-health services, 48
        health-related supportive services, 49
        incentive health plans, 50
        nontraditional services, 50
        value-based payment, 48
Social media, 35
Social network, 14, 34
Social organization, 40
Social Security Act, 49
Social support, 26
Solutions-based approach, 53
Structural change, 41
Sustainability, 20, 41, 43

T
Technology-based interventions
    adolescents and young adults, 33
    effects of, 32

healthcare community, 33
Healthy People 2020, 32
mHealth programs, 33
mobile computing and communication
        technologies, 32
racial/ethnic minority, 32
resource-limited populations, 31
social media, 33, 35
social networks, 33, 34
social sites, 34
telehealth, 35, 36
tele-intensive care unit
        technologies, 35
telemedicine services, 35
Telehealth, 35, 36
Text message reminders, 33
Total Quality Management (TQM), 11
Triple aim of health care, 51
Type I Diabetes, 33

U
Unequal Treatment, 2, 53
United States Department of
        Commerce, 31
United States Department of
        Labor, 25, 26
US Census Bureau, 31
US Department of Health and Human
        Services, 3
US healthcare system, 1

V
Vaccination, 26, 33

W
Workforce diversity, 54

Printed in the United States
By Bookmasters